W9-BNF-373

COMPANION ANIMALS IN HUMAN HEALTH

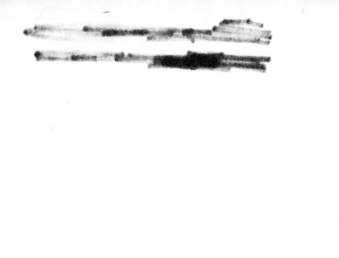

COMPANION ANIMALS IN HUMAN HEALTH

CINDY C. WILSON
DENNIS C. TURNER
EDITORS

SAGE Publications
International Educational and Professional Publisher
Thousand Oaks   London   New Delhi

Copyright © 1998 by Sage Publications, Inc.

All rights reserved. No part of this book may be reproduced or utilized in any form or by any means, electronic or mechanical, including photocopying, recording, or by any information storage and retrieval system, without permission in writing from the publisher.

For information:

SAGE Publications, Inc.
2455 Teller Road
Thousand Oaks, California 91320
E-mail: order@sagepub.com

SAGE Publications Ltd.
6 Bonhill Street
London EC2A 4PU
United Kingdom

SAGE Publications India Pvt. Ltd.
M-32 Market
Greater Kailash I
New Delhi 110 048 India

Printed in the United States of America

Library of Congress Cataloging-in-Publication Data

Main entry under title:

Companion animals in human health / edited by Cindy C. Wilson and
  Dennis C. Turner.
       p.   cm.
    Includes bibliographical references and index.
    ISBN 0-7619-1061-1 (cloth: alk. paper). — ISBN 0-7619-1062-X
(pbk.: alk. paper)
    1. Pets—Therapeutic use.   2. Domestic animals—Therapeutic use.
  I. Wilson, Cindy C.   II. Turner, Dennis C., 1948-   .
  RC931.A65C65   1997
  615.8'515—dc21   98-21077

This book is printed on acid-free paper.

98   99   00   01   02   03   10   9   8   7   6   5   4   3   2   1

Acquiring Editor:	Daniel Ruth
Editorial Assistant:	Anna Howland
Production Editor:	Michele Lingre
Production Assistant:	Denise Santoyo
Typesetter/Designer:	Janelle LeMaster
Indexer:	Cristina Haley
Cover Designer:	Ravi Balasuriya
Print Buyer:	Anna Chin

Contents

Foreword

One day a long time ago, I received a telephone call from "friends of mine" who decided to write and edit a book. They felt somebody (me) should write a preface, or a foreword. Suddenly I found myself staring at over 400 pages of text I was asked to address in just a few pages.

What makes a good preface or foreword in a multi-discipline text? I found a thoughtful one in a book published in 1991 entitled *Man and Beast Revisited,* based in part on a Smithsonian symposium in which I participated. One of the participants in this symposium, Tom Sebeok, recalled that he had been involved in planning and participating in a symposium that was published as a book entitled *Man and Beast: Comparative Social Behavior.* The host for the earlier meeting was, at that time The Smithsonian secretary, S. Dillon Ripley. Sebeok reminded us that Ripley had written a sensitive and richly suggestive preface for this earlier book, justly characterizing it as a "feast of reason." The contributors and editors of this book have not only prepared a feast of reason but a feast of reason and promise.

In 1984, the first meeting of the Delta Society was held at the University of Pennsylvania at the invitation of Aaron Katcher and Alan Beck. During the banquet, the Delta Society announced Boris Levinson and Elizabeth and Sam Corson, as the first recipients of the Delta Distinguished Service award. It was a very happy occasion; and I was privileged to be seated at the same table as the Corsons and Boris Levinson. After the announcement, several people came up to the podium to visit with the honored guests. At this informal get together, Boris Levinson suggested a book be written about the Delta Society and its work. He looked at me and said, "Leo, you should do it."

I was already overextended and there were many within earshot who were well qualified for the task. Many of us had written books in the 80s and 90s, but I knew that none of them filled the voids that Boris addressed. The book which you are now reading comes a long way toward the fulfillment of Boris Levinson's vision.

The Wilson and Turner book challenges us to look beyond the traditional perspective and reevaluate the field of human-animal interactions. For 30 years, attention has been focused upon the human-animal interaction as an all-encompassing rubric for a field of study. What was a seemingly simple relationship with positive outcomes became more complex as researchers and program practitioners collected and analyzed data from various sources. To invoke one of my favorite laws at this juncture: There is no complex problem, which if looked at in the proper way, doesn't become more complex!

Issues arose, including but not limited to: selection of a conceptual framework, accountability for project or program management, credibility with colleagues and institutions, methodology and design, implementation, evaluation, political implications and impact upon professional review, training, training standards, and funding. Other issues related to the multidisciplinary nature of the field and the sometimes, tension provoking relationship between a research and programs. These issues have been both strengths and limitations of the continued development of the field.

As with other clinically related areas, human-animal interaction must use research as the base for program development. At the same time, practitioners must heed the call for documentation and program evaluation in order to focus research endeavors in the most appropriate direction. Research and applied programs co-exist in a mutually interactive state and thus have the unique ability to enhance quality of life assessments by working with each other.

This book, and the works of others, advances the concept of quality of life (QL) as a new perspective for considering, planning, and evaluating new projects, as well as re-evaluating and applying data gathered from older studies and programs. From the overview of potential quality of life outcomes associated with human animal interactions, this book offers the most current research and program interventions in the field. The quality of life construct is developed through critical review of past and existing research outcomes and program interventions. While few quantitative studies have evaluated the impact of a companion animal of quality of life of humans, there is ample evidence to warrant further studies and evaluative projects.

Prior to 1983, there was little scientific evidence to document a measurable association or effect between companion animals and human health. However, between 1990 and 1996, baseline data have outlined applicable information on the use of companion animals as therapeutic interventions. One area of quality of life in which these data are evident is that of social support. This book provides the reader's appreciation of the potential benefits of the various sources of support. Likewise these new studies continue to build the knowledge base while posing essential questions for future endeavors. For example, the nature and value of a strong bond is critical when discussing and comparing effects of interaction of people and animals.

To date, studies have shown animal contact could be healthy, contribute to child development of nurturance and self-concept, promote dialogue among family members, children, people with disabilities, and lonely people, contribute to physiological well-being and improvement of select cardiovascular markers and reduce anxiety levels. However, the combination of these quality of life-enhancing entities was often ignored with the extensive publicity at regional, national, and international levels. Initially this publicity brought well deserved attention to the field of study and programs. However, it became an impediment to the extension of studies on animal assisted therapy. Trained and licensed therapists took exception to considering the use of animals and volunteers to provide therapy, as they are not qualified to do so. Thus, the development of standards is an approach which should help program and research professionals earn the respect of other professional groups.

As a clear definition of variables and outcomes is to applied research studies, a comprehensive set of standards of practice is to animals assisted activities and therapy. Once again, this book offers the reader a feast of information not only on research to date but also the current state-of-the-art for programs.

In its broadest sense, quality of life assessment involves clarification of the values held by an individual, group, or entire society. It may be usefully defined as the process of quantifying human values and incorporating them into important human decisions. If one assumes that quality of life is rooted in individual wants, then one defends the autonomy of individuals so they can define their own concepts of the good life as a form of moral expressions. The question that continues to plague us asks: can any formal assessment take into account individual uniqueness, but still measure quality of life? Perhaps, answers to that question may be found, in part, in the feast of reason that follows.

—Leo K. Bustad

Introduction

Developmentally, the evolution of a field of study can be likened to that of a human (i.e., initially one crawls, walks, and then runs). For the field of human-animal interactions (HAI), growth and development has slowly evolved. From anecdote to pilot study, the field developed increased interest and support from various other disciplines and arenas. From pilot study to experimental design and program evaluation, researchers began to challenge the knowledge base and to test more sophisticated hypotheses against specific conceptual frameworks and paradigms. Data from these studies supplanted anecdote and pilot studies and led to a National Institutes of Health Technology Assessment Workshop in 1987. From this workshop, multi- and interdisciplinary approaches to measuring the therapeutic potential of companion animals on the health of humans was the "step into adolescence." Yet more data were needed to move the field into "adulthood." Explanatory models were needed to serve as a unifying theory base for future work.

Researchers began to publish conceptual models to elicit responses from colleagues and as a means of generating new data and new perspectives; studies became more sophisticated in their approach to assessment of health benefits for both normal and impaired populations. To this end, the Seventh International Conference on Human-Animal Interactions issued its call for papers that looked at HAI on the basis of a conceptual framework of quality of life (QL) for both animals and humans.

The Seventh International Conference, titled "Animals, Health, and Quality of Life," was distinguished by adhering strictly to professionally established criteria for the review of abstracts and subsequent manuscripts. The process, although tedious and time-consuming, resulted in the first blind, peer review conference in this field. Papers presented in Geneva and selected, invited manuscripts were once again submitted to outside review by individuals not involved in this conference or authoring a chapter in this text. These reviewers are well-known in their primary area of research or program evaluation. Once accepted, the manuscripts were also reviewed by the editors, and a great deal of effort went into collaborative and collegial revisions. Although a readily accepted process in most disciplines, this review has focused a great deal of attention on the continued need for strong multidisciplinary and interdisciplinary assessment of research and programs related to HAI.

Interest in QL as a conceptual framework has been stimulated by ethical and financial considerations associated with an aging population and the concomitant increase in chronic illness. QL is applicable, however, to all ages, conditions, and abilities. Broadly defined, QL can be divided into five major constituent domains: (1) physical status and symptoms (includes rest/sleep, energy and vitality, functional abilities, and health perceptions); (2) general life satisfaction; (3) mental/emotional status (includes cognition); (4) social activities; and (5) financial/role activity). Improving QL is a key ingredient in therapeutic interventions as well as in rehabilitation programs; QL is as important to an individual with good health as it is to a person who is hearing impaired or an individual with low self-esteem.

The ways in which QL may be applied in HAI are numerous. QL helps place in context and also delimit the role of HAI. It clarifies that although HAI may affect larger domains of QL, HAI is not solely responsible for doing so. Indeed, its focus of action should be on the determinants and moderators that are most likely to affect health (see chapters in this volume by Collis & McNicholas; Copeland Fitzgerald & Tebay; McNicholas & Collis; Triebenbacher).

The framework can also be used as a checklist for key elements to be considered in developing any therapeutic intervention. It makes clear the macro and immediate environmental, physiologic, and sociopsychological factors that need to be considered along with key moderating factors such as control, opportunities, resources, support systems, and skills.

No longer can the discipline afford small pilot studies as markers in the field. Programs must establish measurable objects, and evaluation criteria must be included, before the scientific community at large will accept the outcomes.

This volume includes perspectives from a wide range of disciplines reflecting both the interest and widely different approaches researchers have taken since the first international conference in the 1970s. Still growing and developing as a discipline, HAI research has yet to define its own theory base and methodologies. Yet the growing maturity of the field is manifested by the obvious attention to the need for strong conceptual frameworks and meticulously applied methodologies. Thus, this volume attempts to link "lessons learned" about HAI and QL with developments of therapeutic interventions and programs to enhance health and well-being.

—Cindy C. Wilson

Acknowledgments

During the production of this book, I have had help from a variety of sources. The contributors have given freely of their time, meeting every request for help. Their help went far beyond professionalism. It spoke volumes of their belief in a field of inquiry that is finally coming into its own. Each has given his or her best effort to improve the field for those who follow and for those whose health is improved and quality of life is enhanced.

It would have been impossible to produce this text without our computer experts. In this day of technology, they made it possible to work internationally without leaving home! They certainly improved my quality of life when they patiently helped me work through one crisis after another. To Stephen R. Brown, Marisa Stoolmiller, and Conan Matthews, who were always ready to answer a "quick question," and to the others at the various institutions who helped me to read, convert, and "talk" between systems— we are indebted to you.

Most of all, my thanks to Jean-Pierre, who made writing this book do-able. For he became the companion for Cable and Zack—all three of whom have made my life fuller and richer because they are part of it.

—*Cindy C. Wilson*

I would like to acknowledge the Swiss Academy of Humanities
and Social Sciences in Berne and the Zurich Animal Protection
for support of my travel to work with Cindy Wilson
in developing the prospectus for the book.

—*Dennis C. Turner*

PART I

Historical and
Value Perspectives

Cindy C. Wilson
Dennis C. Turner

This text challenges us to look beyond our traditional perspectives and reevaluate the field of human-animal interactions. For the past 30 years, much attention has been focused on this term as an all-encompassing rubric for a field of study. What seemingly was a simple relationship with positive outcomes became more complex as researchers and program practitioners evaluated and collected data from various sources. Issues arose that included but were not limited to selection of a conceptual framework, accountability for project or program management, credibility with colleagues and institutions, methodology and design, implementation, evaluation, political implications and impact on professional review, training and training standards, and funding. Other issues relate to the multidisciplinary characteristic of the field and the, sometimes, noncomplementary relationship between research and programs. These two elements have been both the strength and the weakness of the continued development of the field. As with other clinically related areas, human-animal interaction must use its research as a base for program development; at the same time, practitioners must heed the call for documentation and program evaluations to focus research endeavors in the most appropriate direction. Research and programs coexist in a mutually interactive state and thus have the unique ability to enhance quality of life assessments by working with each other.

This text advances the concept of *quality of life* (QL) as a new perspective for considering, planning, and evaluating new projects as well as reevaluating and applying data gathered from older studies and programs. Part I provides an overview and potential QL outcomes of the work to date in research (Garrity & Stallones), animal-assisted therapy programs (Hines & Fredrickson) and hippotherapy and therapeutic riding (Copeland Fitzpatrick & Tebay). A critical review of past and existing research outcomes and program interventions is key in determining whether we can meet the challenge to the field to document the therapeutic value of animal intervention.

Effects of Pet Contact on Human Well-Being 1

Review of Recent Research

Thomas F. Garrity
Lorann Stallones

Abstract

Contact with companion animals has been hypothesized to enhance the quality of life of their human partners. A search of the scientific literature between 1990 and 1995 uncovered 25 empirical studies in the English language addressing this issue. Using the social support paradigm derived from the human well-being literature, the 25 studies were examined according to types of support offered, types of models tested, and types of well-being affected. In addition, studies are analyzed by types of research design employed. The review concludes that although research progress continues to be slow in this area, findings of quality of life benefits derived from companion animal contact are consistent with the research reported during the past two decades in the literature on human social support. These benefits are evident on the psychological, physical, social, and behavioral levels. The quality of life benefits of pet association, however, are apparent only in certain situations and under certain circumstances.

Introduction

Reviews of the literature provide status reports on progress in busy fields of scientific research. The literature on companion animal effects on human health and psychosocial well-being has regularly benefited from such reviews (Barba, 1995; Baun, Oetting, & Bergstrom, 1991; Beck & Katcher, 1984; Boldt & Dellmann-Jenkins, 1992; Edney, 1992; Felthous & Kellert, 1987; Mallon, 1992; Patronek & Glickman, 1993; Rowan & Beck, 1994). In addition, a bibliography of articles published from 1983 to 1990 has been compiled by the National Library of Medicine, titled Human-Pet Relationships (Hunt, 1991). A common conclusion of these reviews was that quantitative studies that document the role of companion animals in the relationships assessed were rare. There was also general agreement that certain areas had sufficient evidence to warrant further study.

Prior to 1983, published scientific literature contained little evidence to document a measurable association between pet contact and human health. Generalizable inferences could not be made because of limited use of conceptual models and because of methodological shortcomings (Marx, 1984).

Between 1983 and 1989, however, a number of studies appeared that addressed relationships between human well-being and the presence of companion animals in households. Using a quality of life conceptual framework, this chapter reviews and examines research productivity from 1990 to 1995.

Review of Literature, 1990 to 1995

Plan of Search

This literature review examines published empirical studies of the physical, psychological, social, and other behavioral effects of contacts with companion animals on the humans with whom they interact. Three clusters of research are excluded from the following review. First, research with a child development perspective that examines relationships between pet contact and contemporaneous or later personality effects is excluded. The second excluded cluster is that on the use of animals as therapeutic adjuncts to medical or psychiatric therapy. A third cluster that is excluded deals with the bereavement experiences of people who have lost pets to death. These deletions result from our primary interest in a theoretical perspective described in the following paragraph.

Within the companion animal-human bond literature exists a sizable group of studies that appear to spring from a preexisting paradigm relating human social support to aspects of human well-being. Social scientists have long postulated and studied the benefits that accrue to people who receive social, emotional, material, and informational benefits from other people. Given the obvious subjective satisfaction and assistance received from pets, it was natural that biobehavioral researchers would eventually wish to study systematically the existence, nature, and extent of the benefits of pet contact for people. In this perspective, pets are viewed as a type of nonhuman social support capable of conferring health and behavioral benefits on their human partners.

The literature review was conducted using the National Library of Medicine's MedLine database and the American Psychological Association's PsycLIT database for calendar years 1990 through 1995. Additional searches of ERIC and CINAHL databases provided no additional articles to those already identified in MedLine and PsycLIT. Dissertation abstracts were examined, but the decision was made to include only published articles because they are most likely to have been subjected to external peer review. Review articles from both the 1990-1995 and earlier periods were also carefully examined and are commented on in this chapter, but only data-based, empirical articles were subjected to analysis. Only English-language citations were included in this review. Searches were conducted on key words *pets* and *companion animals.*

Yield of Search

Twenty-five articles met the criteria of our search. More than a hundred citations were initially identified; the majority were excluded because they did not deal with the biobehavioral effects of pet contact on humans. Many others were excluded: editorials and commentaries (e.g., Hart, Hart, & Mader, 1990; Rowan & Beck, 1994), program descriptions (e.g., Lapp, 1991), therapeutic trials of pets in medical practice (e.g., Draper, Gerber, & Layng, 1990), and literature reviews (e.g., Boldt & Dellmann-Jenkins, 1992; Patronek & Glickman, 1993). Reviewed articles were drawn from 12 periodicals, but the majority were found in just 4: *Anthrozoös* (7), *Psychological Reports* (4), *Journal of Nervous and Mental Disease* (2), and *Journal of Personality and Social Psychology* (2). All studies included adult study participants; one, however, included a few children in a predominantly adult sample (Loughlin & Dowrick, 1993), and one examined parent-child dyads (Cox, 1993). Five studies were drawn from selected populations of patients (e.g., HIV [Carmack, 1991] and infertility [Blenner, 1991]), 6 were of older, generally well adults, and 12 included younger, well adults. In the studies of patients, pets were viewed as providing general social support rather than specific input to medical therapy.

Orientation to Social Support Paradigm

Research on human-animal interactions is related to, and perhaps springs from, the research tradition on social support received from other people. Two aspects of human social support research have dominated conceptual discussion; these also have relevance for research in the companion animal realm.

Types of Social Support

In the human social support literature, distinctions have been made between the types of support offered by other people. Support may be aids such as money, shelter, or transportation. Support may be emotional, with expressions of sympathy and esteem for and confidence in the recipient. Informational support may take the form of advice and consultation that enables the recipient to formulate additional ways of appraising and coping with challenging situations. In addition, the human research on social support has approached measurement in ways that suggest distinct types of support. One approach involves a structural concept in which social linkages to other people are counted; a second approach assesses the subjective quality of the support as appraised by the recipient.

The research examined for this review indicates that the pet support literature is still using more rudimentary conceptual and operational definitions of support than in the more advanced human support field. Of the 25 articles we reviewed, 14 take a structural approach to pet support measurement, namely, pet ownership compared with nonownership, or simple contact with pets compared with noncontact (Allen, Blascovich, Tomaka, & Kelsey, 1991; Anderson, Reid, & Jennings, 1992; Blenner,

1991; Carmack, 1991; DeSchriver & Riddick, 1990; Hirsch & Whitman, 1994; Loughlin & Dowrick, 1993; Miller, Staats, & Partlo, 1992; Nielsen & Delude, 1994; Peretti, 1990; Rogers, Hart, & Boltz, 1993; Serpell, 1991; Straede & Gates, 1993; Wilson, 1991). This approach is analogous to the assessment of the availability of a confidant in the human literature and is certainly not without value, as a large literature on the health benefits of social connectedness attests (Cohen & Syme, 1985). The somewhàt more sophisticated qualitative approach that measures the subjective nature and meaning of social contacts also has its counterpart in the pet support literature. It is represented by studies that use indicators of the intensity of attachment to pets. Three of the reviewed studies take the attachment approach exclusively (Cox, 1993; St. Yves, Freeston, Jacques, & Robitaille, 1990; Tucker, Friedman, Tsai, & Martin, 1995), and an additional eight use both the qualitative attachment and the structural approaches (Friedmann, Locker, & Lockwood, 1993; Fritz, Farver, Kass, & Hart, 1995; Kidd & Kidd, 1994; Loyer-Carlson, 1992; Siegel, 1990; Stallones, Marx, Garrity, & Johnson, 1990; Watson & Weinstein, 1993; Zasloff & Kidd, 1994).

In the other aspects of support (i.e., material, emotional, and informational), none of the studies ventured into that realm for predicting effects. Animals, by their nature, can offer a smaller range of types of support than can people but still offer a rich mix of possible types of benefit. One article surveyed bird owners to assess the reasons for owning this type of pet (Loughlin & Dowrick, 1993). Reasons included giving and receiving love, companionship, security, feeling needed, adding to the meaning of life, and others. The study is one of the few that look more closely at types of social support offered by pets, but it did not attempt to relate these types of support to other variables such as aspects of well-being.

These observations suggest possibilities for extension of future research. First, operationalization of the pet factor as simple ownership compared with nonownership neglects the importance of other aspects of pet support. Better approaches would involve objective and subjective measurements of types of support represented by ownership or simple contact. The use of measures of attachment is now fairly common yet is still seen in a minority of the studies reviewed. Rarer still are efforts to identify types of support derived from pet contact and studies of possible differences these might make for humans. Less common as well in both pet and human studies of support are studies of "negative support" derived from pets and its effects on human well-being. This represents the sorts of difficulties, threats, obstructions, and socioemotional hassles deriving from other people and pets. It is not surprising that research on negative support is not common when both human and animal literatures typically start with the assumption that support is generally health-promoting and protective. Pets may be seen as increasing the problems of life, however, rather than alleviating them; animal bites and allergens have received attention in the literature and do have obvious effects on human well-being. Research in this area would profit from attempts to clarify pet support effects in positive and negative directions.

Models of Social Support

One model of the influence of social support, the direct effect view, simply portrays social support as having an unmediated, direct impact on aspects of human well-being. The well-known Alameda County data of Berkman and Syme (1979), for example, indicate in a prospective epidemiological design that involvement in supportive human social relationships is associated with enhanced survival during a 9-year follow-up. Although survival benefits springing from social support may be at least partially mediated by other factors, it appears that human support in its own right affects the outcome as well.

In the pet support literature reviewed, the direct effects model was the overwhelming choice of models guiding research. Of the 25 articles, 17 reviewed employed only the direct effects model (Anderson et al., 1992; Cox, 1993; DeSchriver & Riddick, 1990; Fritz et al., 1995; Hirsch & Whitman, 1994; Loughlin & Dowrick, 1993; Loyer-Carlson, 1992; Miller et al., 1992; Nielsen & Delude, 1994; Rogers et al., 1993; Serpell, 1991; Straede & Gates, 1993; St. Yves et al., 1990; Tucker et al., 1995; Watson & Weinstein, 1993; Wilson, 1991; Zasloff & Kidd, 1994). Watson and Weinstein (1993), for example, hypothesized that working women who owned cats and/or dogs would experience less emotional distress (depression, anxiety, and anger) than nonowners; those owners who were more attached to their pets were expected to experience less emotional distress. Although neither of these hypotheses were supported in their results, the underlying model was one of direct effect. Straede and Gates (1993) hypothesized that adult cat owners would be psychologically healthier than nonowners. In this study, nonowners were indeed found to report more symptoms of psychological ill health, measured with the General Health

Questionnaire (Goldberg, 1972). Again, the underlying model is that of direct effect between ownership and psychological symptoms.

The alternative model is referred to as the *buffering model* (Cohen & McKay, 1984). This model views social support as somehow intervening to protect the individual from damage to well-being when the person is under siege from stressful life events. In this model, social support operates protectively when the individual is threatened by life stress; in situations of low stress, social support is viewed as unrelated to well-being. The older study of Nuckolls, Cassel, and Kaplan (1972) offers an example of the buffering perspective in the human support literature. Measures of recent life events, human social supports, and complications of pregnancy were obtained from 177 white primipara patients cared for at the same medical center obstetric service. Although neither life events nor social support independently predicted the incidence of medical complications, in combination, prediction followed the model: 91% of the patients with high life stress before and during pregnancy and low social supports experienced complications of their pregnancies. Only 33% of their high stress-high social support counterparts experienced complications, indicating that the presence of a variety of assistance from spouses, families, and friends lessens the strain induced by significant life challenges. Only 46% of patients without such a history of stressful life events, regardless of social support level, had pregnancy complications. The latter result may indicate that adequate social support becomes an advantage for health status only when the person is engaged in a struggle to adapt to the challenging changes of life.

Of the 25 articles on pet support reviewed, only 6 included a buffering perspective (Allen et al., 1991; Blenner, 1991; Carmack, 1991; Friedmann et al., 1993; Siegel, 1990; Stallones et al., 1990). Siegel hypothesized that in a prospective study, pet ownership would be associated with fewer physician contacts among male and female Medicare beneficiaries who belong to a large California health maintenance organization. Using the direct effect model, pet ownership significantly predicted physician contacts in the expected direction after adjustment for a variety of other factors. Using the buffering effect model, it was found that among participants with more life events stress, pet owners saw the doctor less often than nonowners during the 1-year follow-up. Among participants with less life events stress, physician contacts were comparable, thereby approximating the expected configuration of results in the buffering model. These pet support effects were found among dog owners but not among owners of cats and birds. Secondary analysis indicated that this may result from greater attachment and interactions between dogs and their owners than between other types of animals and their owners.

Stallones and colleagues (1990) provide a second example of inclusion of the buffering perspective. Following their earlier results in a national study of older pet owners and nonowners (Garrity, Stallones, Marx, & Johnson, 1989), they hypothesized that in three age categories from 21 through 64 years, pet owners (compared with nonowners) and owners who were more attached to pets (compared with those less attached) would experience advantages in several aspects of well-being. The buffering perspective emerges as pet effects on well-being are examined at various levels of negative life changes. Neither pet factor proved to be significantly related to any measure of human well-being in any of the three age groups. Pet factors demonstrated no independent effects either as direct or buffering influences on human well-being. These negative results in younger adults contrast with several interesting pet benefits found among older persons (Garrity et al., 1989).

A third example of the buffering model is found in the work of Allen and colleagues (1991). In a complex experimental design, adult women owners of dogs worked on stressful mental arithmetic tasks in the psychophysiology laboratory and at home. In the latter setting, some were randomized to work on the arithmetic tasks in the presence of their own pet dogs, some in the presence of their best female friend, and some in the control condition with only the experimenter present. Results indicated that physiological arousal (skin conductance, blood pressure, and pulse rate) in those accompanied by a friend was significantly greater than in those in the control condition. In turn, arousal was significantly greater in the control condition than in the pet-present condition. In keeping with the buffering paradigm, it appeared that the presence of a pet during acute stress lessened the physiological consequences of stress; to the contrary, human support, in this stressful situation, actually potentiated the physiological strain. As the buffering model predicts, there were no differences among conditions (i.e., friend present, pet present, and control) in the low-stress rest periods between arithmetic tasks. The authors interpreted the results as the nonevaluative nature of pet support compared with human support. In this situation, human presence may be an example of negative support discussed earlier.

Although neither conceptual approach—direct effect nor buffering—is inherently superior, investigators in the pet support field may be able to enrich their studies by considering both models as they plan their work. It appears that with the addition of measures of stressful life conditions and statistical analyses that test buffering relationships (Baron & Kenny, 1986), some direct effects projects could add considerable useful data on ways in which pets might influence human well-being. Few of the reviewed articles examine pet contact as a buffer, whereas in much of the current and older literature, pet contact is discussed as a source of comfort and protection in a difficult and challenging world.

Research Design

Research designs range from approaches that explore and describe, which are fruitful for generating hypotheses for testing in more fully controlled types of design, to controlled experimental designs that offer greater possibilities for demonstrating causal connections between variables of interest. Toward the middle of the continuum are found designs that attempt to test hypotheses about associations among variables, but without the ability of demonstrating definitively that variables are causally related. In this section, we will describe the research literature from 1990 through 1995 in relation to the research designs employed.

Descriptive Research

Four of the 25 studies reviewed are descriptive and exploratory in nature. The project of Loughlin and Dowrick (1993) entailed the compilation of a list of human psychological needs fulfilled by owning birds. Data were derived from responses to a questionnaire by a convenience sample of 80 bird owners ranging in age from 9 years to 82 years. The questionnaire contained 36 statements reflecting possible reasons for owning birds that might be endorsed by respondents. The resulting list might provide useful ideas for further, more systematic testing of hypotheses about links between motivations for pet ownership and benefits derived from them. The previously mentioned studies of Blenner (1991) and Carmack (1991) also fall in this category. The former interviewed pet-owning infertile couples undergoing treatment, and the latter interviewed patients with HIV/AIDS infections to identify the benefits of pet ownership in coping with their medical conditions. Again, these descriptive results might provide insights leading to more rigorously controlled investigations and intervention programs using pets in facilitating treatment and patient adjustment. Finally, Peretti (1990) gathered open-ended statements from older men and women on motivations for owning dogs. Five principal reasons in men and women were listed and compared.

Correlational Research

Of the 25 studies, 16 were correlational in that two or more variables were examined in light of hypotheses that postulate associations of some sort (Anderson et al., 1992; Cox, 1993; Fritz et al., 1995; Hirsch & Whitman, 1994; Kidd & Kidd, 1994; Loyer-Carlson, 1992; Miller et al., 1992; Rogers et al., 1993; Serpell, 1991; Siegel, 1990; Stallones et al., 1990; Straede & Gates, 1993; St. Yves et al., 1990; Tucker et al., 1995; Watson & Weinstein, 1993; Zasloff & Kidd, 1994). Most of these projects were cross-sectional in relation to the timing of data collection. Three (Serpell, 1991; Siegel, 1990; Tucker et al., 1995), however, took a more advanced approach by measuring variables longitudinally. This approach enables analysis that provides a better assessment of temporal and perhaps causal ordering of key variables.

The work of Hirsch and Whitman (1994) exemplifies the cross-sectional, correlational design. The investigators hypothesized that social support from pets and/or people in the household would confer preventive benefits to the afflictions of headaches and chronic pain of other sources. Using the "case-control" approach, Hirsch and Whitman found that patients with headaches and chronic pain problems were as likely to have pets and household members living with them as were patients without problems of headache and pain. Hence, contrary to hypothesis, pet and human supports as measured in this study were not associated with protection from problems of headache and various types of chronic pain. In a study not guided by specific hypotheses, Miller et al. (1992) sought to identify characteristics of older (50 to 92 years), mostly female (75%) individuals associated with the likelihood of interacting with pets. Correlations, not necessarily causal, were found between interacting with pets and better perceived health, younger age, more education, having more children at home, experiencing more daily hassles and uplifts, greater satisfaction with life, and more positive expectations for the future. Pet interactors who derive more uplifts from their pets were also found to engage in more social interaction with other people, for example, talking with friends and doing things with friends. As with all correlational research, caution must be observed not to conclude that relationships found between variables are necessarily causal. In this study, for example, some third variable such as health status may explain both pet interaction variables and their correlates (e.g., positive expectations for the future).

Siegel's (1990) study is an example of a correlational study that measures key variables longitudinally rather than cross-sectionally. Most key predictor variables were queried before the major outcome variable. Hence, measures of stress, pet and human social support, and demographic factors were asked at baseline, whereas the measurement of the health outcome (i.e., contacts with physicians) was done longitudinally at 2-month intervals for a year. The major advantage of such a research design is the ability to establish temporal ordering and to control for the influence of earlier levels of key outcome variables. Tucker and colleagues (1995) provide another example of the longitudinal, correlational approach. Using a data set initiated in 1921, new information about extent of play with pets was collected in 1977 from more than 600 men and women with an average age of 67 years. Although pet contact did not relate to survival through 1991, the longitudinal design did enable the investigators to establish clear temporal separation between predictor variables and outcome. In this study, the longitudinal design does present a problem in establishing whether pet support continued to be available to the participants from 1977 until close to the time of death; data were simply not available on this issue after 1977. This weakens the conclusions that can be drawn regarding possible benefits of pet support for survival in older persons.

Experimental Research

Five of the 25 studies reviewed were experimental in nature (Allen et al., 1991; DeSchriver & Riddick, 1990; Friedmann et al., 1993; Nielsen & Delude, 1994; Wilson, 1991). They entailed introduction of an experimental manipulation in a setting in which some important potentially confounding factors have been controlled; these designs are referred to as quasi-experimental designs. Allen and coworkers (1991) introduced a pet or best friend support as compared with a control condition. The carefully described experimental situation could be controlled to only a limited extent because it took place in the home setting of the participants. Although this limits the level of control possible, it enhances the external validity by using a largely naturalistic setting. The study of Wilson (1991) is another example of quasi-experimental design. Young adult college student volunteers who were predominantly white women provided data on their state and trait anxiety (Spielberger, Gorsuch, & Lushene, 1970) in three experimental conditions: reading aloud, reading quietly, and petting a friendly but unknown dog. The manipulations, represented by the three conditions, affected state anxiety overall, such that reading aloud generated higher scores than reading quietly and petting the dog, which produced similar levels of state anxiety.

Although types of research designs range along continuum from descriptive to experimental designs, it would be wrong to conclude that the former designs are of lesser scientific value than the latter. Carefully conducted and theoretically informed descriptive research can make important scientific contributions, whereas poorly conceived and conducted quasi-experiments can be scientifically worthless.

The predominance of the correlational designs does raise questions about why they are so prevalent. Correlational studies, especially those that are cross-sectional, permit the collection of data on a large number of variables in a relatively short time, and at a relatively low cost. Hence, many variables can be measured using questionnaires and behavioral checklists that can be completed in a short time. Longitudinal, correlational designs share some of these economies but add the costs of more than a single point of contact with participants through time.

Types of Well-Being Examined

The 25 studies reviewed exhibited four types of well-being that were of primary interest: psychological, social, behavioral, and physiological or physical health indicators of human well-being. These elements were likely chosen because of their impact on the quality of life of participants.

Psychological

Ten of these articles examined only psychological indicators of well-being (Blenner, 1991; Carmack, 1991; Fritz et al., 1995; Miller et al., 1992; Peretti, 1990; Straede & Gates, 1993; St. Yves et al., 1990; Watson & Weinstein, 1993; Wilson, 1991; Zasloff & Kidd, 1994); three additional projects examined psychological and other measures of well-being (Loughlin & Dowrick, 1993; Serpell, 1991; Stallones et al., 1990). Zasloff and Kidd (1994) identified loneliness, measured by the Revised UCLA Loneliness Scale (Russell, Peplau, & Cutrona, 1980), as their sole indicator of well-being. In this study of women college students, this psychological variable was found no different between pet owners and nonowners and no different between less and more highly attached owners. They did find, however, that participants living entirely alone were more lonely than those living with either pet alone, pets and people, or people alone. The study of St. Yves and colleagues (1990) provides another example of use of a psychological indicator of well-being, measures of wanted and expressed interpersonal affection (Schutz, 1966). In this sample of 149 adults from Quebec City, the hypothesis that love for animals (Ray, 1982) would be related to both expression of and desire for interpersonal affection was not supported.

Social

Three of 25 studies focused exclusively on social indicators of well-being (Cox, 1993; Loyer-Carlson, 1992; Nielsen & Delude, 1994); an additional three examined social and another type of well-being (Loughlin & Dowrick, 1993; Rogers et al., 1993; Stallones et al., 1990). Loyer-Carlson (1992), for example, employed a measure of perceived quality of family life. This measured the respondent's evaluation of the quality of six interpersonal resources exchanged in family relationships, such as love, services, and information (Rettig, Danes, & Bauer, 1989). Analysis failed to demonstrate a relationship between pet presence in the family or pet bonding (Poresky, Hendrix, Mosier, & Samuelson, 1987) and family life quality. Liking pets (Poresky, Hendrix, Mosier, & Samuelson, 1988), however, was found to correlate moderately with family life quality. A second study (Cox, 1993) that focused exclusively on social well-being in which the relationships of pet attachment, measured with the Pet Attachment Scale (Templer, Salter, Dickey, Baldwin, & Veleber, 1981), and family adaptability and family cohesion, measured with the FACES III (Olson, Portner, & Lavee, 1985), were examined. Although significant correlations were found between pet attachment and both measures of family functioning, generalizability remains a question because the study sample reflected a low response rate from a population of unknown characteristics.

Behavioral

Six of the 25 studies included behavioral measures of well-being (Allen et al., 1991; Rogers et al., 1993; Serpell, 1991; Siegel, 1990; Stallones et al., 1990; Tucker et al., 1995). Rogers et al., 1993 examined behaviors associated with walking with and without pet dogs among a small sample of older people living in a mobile home park. Dog walkers walked more frequently than those who had no dogs; median time spent walking during each walk was comparable in the two groups. Other measures of social, emotional, and health well-being derived from the Duke University Older Americans Resource Survey (Duke University Center for Study of Aging and Human Development, 1978) suggested a well-being advantage for the dog walkers. Again, the small sample size raises questions about generalizability of results. The earlier described experimental study of Allen and coworkers (1991) examined the effects of pet or friend presence on performance of arithmetic calculations. This behavioral indicator of well-being showed a clear advantage in favor of pet presence over that of a friend. Finally, Tucker and colleagues (1995) examined associations between reports of "playing with pets" and the propensity to engage in health-promoting behaviors. They found no differences between those older participants with and without this sort of pet contact.

Physical

Physiological or physical health measures of well-being were used in 7 of the 25 studies reviewed (Allen et al., 1991; Anderson et al., 1992; DeSchriver & Riddick, 1990; Friedmann et al., 1993; Hirsch & Whitman, 1994; Serpell, 1991; Tucker et al., 1995). Allen and colleagues (1991) subjected participants to stressful mental arithmetic tasks with pet, close human friend, or neither present. Measures of autonomic arousal (skin conductance, blood pressure, and pulse rate) were recorded. Autonomic reactivity was consistently greatest in the friend condition, which was significantly greater than control condition, which in turn was significantly greater than pet condition. Anderson and colleagues (1992) examined various cardiovascular risk factors in pet owners and nonowners; they found advantages in systolic blood pressure, serum cholesterol, and triglyceride in men who were pet owners in comparison with their non-owner counterparts. Pet owners also exercised more than nonowners.

Psychological indicators tend to predominate as measures of human well-being in the recent studies reviewed. In addition to the importance of psychological variables, cost and convenience issues help to explain this situation. Whereas psychological variables can usually be measured using simple and relatively inexpensive questionnaires completed by the study participants, measures of physiological responses require more or less complicated electronic equipment, and behavioral and illness measures may require labor-intense observations or records searches. Psychological factors also have a variety of already validated scales available for measuring a variety of emotional states. Nonetheless, the predominance of studies on psychological effects may suggest a direction for further work. Certainly, there is still much room for well-designed studies of pet effects in relation to physical health and physiological status. Studies of personal and social behaviors of many types have been relatively neglected in the recent literature.

Results: Pet Supports and Well-Being

At the most general level, 16 of the 25 studies reported at least some advantage in having contact with companion animals (Allen et al., 1991; Anderson et al., 1992; Blenner, 1991; Carmack, 1991; Cox, 1993; Friedmann et al., 1993; Fritz et al., 1995; Loyer-Carlson, 1992; Miller et al., 1992; Nielsen & Delude, 1994; Rogers et al., 1993; Serpell, 1991; Siegel, 1990; Straede & Gates, 1993; Wilson, 1991; Zasloff & Kidd, 1994). We must also report, however, that 11 of these 25 studies reported at least partial negative results, that is, pet contact conferred no advantage for well-being (DeSchriver & Riddick, 1990; Fritz et al., 1995; Hirsch & Whitman, 1994; Loyer-Carlson, 1992; Stallones et al., 1990; Straede &

Gates, 1993; St. Yves et al., 1990; Tucker et al., 1995; Watson & Weinstein, 1993; Wilson, 1991; Zasloff & Kidd, 1994). This is a considerable proportion of negative results, considering the well-known bias toward submitting and publishing results that support the hypotheses of the researchers. In addition, even this picture is too simple because it does not factor in an evaluation of the methodological rigor of the reviewed research.

Although a relatively small number of studies spanning the 1990 to 1995 period were reviewed, there was a great variety of variables studied. This makes generalization about consistencies in the results difficult. Even in those few instances in which there was similarity of variables from study to study, and even with the same measurement, there are difficulties in generalizing results. For example, 11 studies examined psychological indicators of well-being. Among these studies, the most frequently examined variable was anxiety, included in 4 (Fritz et al., 1995; Straede & Gates, 1993; Watson & Weinstein, 1993; Wilson, 1991) of the 11. Three of these four measured anxiety with the Spielberger State-Trait Anxiety Inventory (Spielberger et al., 1970). One study found anxiety (measured by caregiver reports) significantly lower in Alzheimer patients who were exposed to pets than in those not exposed to pets (Fritz et al., 1995). Two other studies found anxiety (measured by the Spielberger state inventory) unrelated to pet ownership (Straede & Gates, 1993; Watson & Weinstein, 1993). The fourth study found Spielberger's state anxiety score significantly lower in those petting a dog than in those reading aloud; the same study found that there was no difference in state anxiety between those petting a dog and those reading quietly (Wilson, 1991). The only other construct in which there is overlap in variable selection and measurement is with depression, examined in four articles (Fritz et al., 1995; Stallones et al., 1990; Straede & Gates, 1993; Watson & Weinstein, 1993), with the Beck Depression Inventory (Beck, 1987) used in two of the four. None of these four studies demonstrates a significant relationship between pet exposure and depression. This cluster of results demonstrates the difficulties in generalizing from the recent literature. Hence, in the more recent literature, support for the notion that pet contact is related to less anxiety or depression is minimal and contradictory.

In addition to the heterogeneity of variables of interest and approaches to measurement, difficulty in generalizing findings may also be ascribed to differences in populations being studied. The 25 studies were nearly equally divided among focuses on young adults, older persons, and patient groups with a variety of illness problems. Sample sizes ranged from fewer than 10 (Nielsen & Delude, 1994) to more than 5,500 (Anderson et al., 1992). Study designs were quite variable; generalizations about pet effects are not yet possible.

These cautions notwithstanding, there appears to be sufficient evidence in the studies appearing since 1990 to warrant several tentative conclusions. First, benefits from contacts with pets seem generally consistent with the benefits already strongly supported by research through two decades in human social support. Second, in relation to pets, these benefits probably occur on the psychological, physical, social, and behavioral levels. Third, the benefits of pet association are apparent only in certain situations and under certain circumstances. Identification of these special moderating influences should occupy a major portion of future research in this area. Fourth, pet association probably benefits a person both directly and as a protective or buffering factor when the person is threatened by life circumstances.

These promising directions will require more attention than they have received in the past 5 years. With only 25 studies identified during this period, it is clear that advances in the understanding of pets as supports to human well-being are proceeding too slowly. Additional trained biobehavioral scientists are needed to work in this area. Incentives are needed and will surely advance this cause. Continued and, perhaps, expanded support from industrial sources and opportunistic inclusion in governmentally sponsored projects may provide the engine that will move researchers forward more rapidly in this enterprise.

References

Allen, K. M., Blascovich, J., Tomaka, J., & Kelsey, R. M. (1991). Presence of human friends and pet dogs as moderators of autonomic responses to stress in women. *Journal of Personality and Social Psychology, 61,* 582-589.

Anderson, W. P., Reid, C. M., & Jennings, G. L. (1992). Pet ownership and risk factors for cardiovascular disease. *Medical Journal of Australia, 157,* 298-301.

Barba, B. E. (1995). A critical review of research on the human/companion animal relationship: 1988 to 1993. *Anthrozoös, 8,* 9-15.

Baron, R. M., & Kenny, D. A. (1986). The moderator-mediator variable distinction in social psychological research: Conceptual, strategic, and statistical considerations. *Journal of Personality and Social Psychology, 51,* 1173-1182.

Baun, M. M., Oetting, K., & Bergstrom, N. (1991). Health benefits of companion animals in relation to the physiologic indices of relaxation. *Holistic Nursing Practice, 5,* 16-23.

Beck, A. M., & Katcher, A. H. (1984). A new look at pet-facilitated therapy. *Journal of the American Veterinary Medical Association, 184,* 414-421.

Beck, A. T. (1987). *Beck depression inventory manual.* San Antonio, TX: Psychological Corporation.

Berkman, L. F., & Syme, S. L. (1979). Host resistance and mortality: A nine-year follow-up study of Alameda County residents. *American Journal of Epidemiology, 109,* 186-204.

Blenner, J. L. (1991). The therapeutic functions of companion animals in infertility. *Holistic Nursing Practice, 5,* 6-10.

Boldt, M. A., & Dellmann-Jenkins, M. (1992). The impact of companion animals in later life and considerations for practice. *Journal of Applied Gerontology, 11,* 228-239.

Carmack, B. J. (1991). The role of companion animals for persons with AIDS/HIV. *Holistic Nursing Practice, 5,* 24-31.

Cohen, S., & McKay, G. (1984). Social support, stress, and the buffering hypothesis: A theoretical analysis. In A. Baum, J. E. Singer, & S. E. Taylor (Eds.), *Handbook of psychology and health* (Vol. 4, pp. 253-267). Hillsdale, NJ: Lawrence Erlbaum.

Cohen, S., & Syme, S. L. (Eds.). (1985). *Social support and health.* New York: Academic Press.

Cox, R. P. (1993). The human/animal bond as a correlate of family functioning. *Clinical Nursing Research, 2,* 222-231.

DeSchriver, M. M., & Riddick, C. C. (1990). Effects of watching aquariums on elders' stress. *Anthrozoös, 4,* 44-48.

Draper, R. J., Gerber, G. J., & Layng, E. M. (1990). Defining the role of pet animals in psychotherapy. *Psychiatric Journal of the University of Ottawa, 15,* 169-172.

Duke University Center for Study of Aging and Human Development. (1978). *Multidimensional functional assessment: The OARS methodology* (2nd ed.). Durham, NC: Duke University Press.

Edney, A. T. B. (1992). Companion animals and human health. *Veterinary Record, 130,* 285-287.

Felthous, A. R., & Kellert, S. R. (1987). Childhood cruelty to animals and alter aggression against people: A review. *American Journal of Psychiatry, 144,* 710-717.

Friedmann, E., Locker, B. Z., & Lockwood, R. (1993). Perception of animals and cardiovascular responses during verbalization with an animal present. *Anthrozoös, 6,* 115-134.

Fritz, C. L., Farver, T. B., Kass, P. H., & Hart, L. A. (1995). Association with companion animals and the expression of non-cognitive symptoms in Alzheimer's patients. *Journal of Nervous and Mental Disease, 183,* 459-463.

Garrity, T. F., Stallones, L., Marx, M. B., & Johnson, T. P. (1989). Pet ownership and attachment as supportive factors in the health of the elderly. *Anthrozoös, 3,* 35-44.

Goldberg, D. P. (1972). *The detection of psychiatric illness by questionnaire.* London: Oxford University Press.

Hart, L. A., Hart, B. L., & Mader, B. (1990). Humane euthanasia and companion animal death: Caring for the animal, the client, and the veterinarian. *Journal of the American Veterinary Medical Association, 197,* 1292-1299.

Hirsch, A. R., & Whitman, B. W. (1994). Pet ownership and prophylaxis of headache and chronic pain. *Headache, 34,* 542-543.

Hunt, J. (1991). *Human-pet relationships: January 1983 through December 1990.* Bethesda, MD: U.S. Department of Health and Human Services.

Kidd, A. H., & Kidd, R. M. (1994). Benefits and liabilities of pets for the homeless. *Psychological Reports, 74,* 715-722.

Lapp, C. A. (1991). Nursing students and the elderly: Enhancing intergenerational communication through human-animal interaction. *Holistic Nursing Practice, 5,* 72-79.

Loughlin, C. A., & Dowrick, D. W. (1993). Psychological needs filled by avian companions. *Anthrozoös, 6,* 166-172.

Loyer-Carlson, V. (1992). Pets and perceived family life quality. *Psychological Reports, 70,* 947-952.

Mallon, G. P. (1992). Utilization of animals as therapeutic adjuncts with children and youth: A review of the literature. *Child and Youth Care Forum, 21,* 53-67.

Marx, M. B. (1984). The salubrious endearment: Review of "New perspectives on our lives with companion animals." *Contemporary Psychology, 29,* 902-903.

Miller, D., Staats, S., & Partlo, C. (1992). Discriminating positive and negative aspects of pet interaction: Sex differences in the older population. *Social Indicators Research, 27,* 363-374.

Nielsen, J. A., & Delude, L. A. (1994). Pets as adjunct therapists in a residence for former psychiatric patients. *Anthrozoös, 7,* 166-171.

Nuckolls, K. B., Cassel, J., & Kaplan, B. H. (1972). Psychosocial assets, life crisis, and the prognosis of pregnancy. *American Journal of Epidemiology, 95,* 431-444.

Olson, D., Portner, J., & Lavee, Y. (1985). *FACES III: Family social science.* St. Paul: University of Minnesota Press.

Patronek, G. J., & Glickman, L. T. (1993). Pet ownership protects against the risks and consequences of coronary heart disease. *Medical Hypotheses, 40,* 245-249.

Peretti, P. O. (1990). Elderly-animal friendship bonds. *Social Behavior and Personality, 18,* 151-156.

Poresky, R. H., Hendrix, C., Mosier, J. E., & Samuelson, M. L. (1987). The Companion Animal Bonding Scale: Internal reliability and construct validity. *Psychological Reports, 60,* 743-746.

Poresky, R. H., Hendrix, C., Mosier, J. E., & Samuelson, M. L. (1988). The Companion Animal Semantic Differential: Long and short form reliability and validity. *Educational and Psychological Measurement, 48,* 255-260.

Ray, J. J. (1982). Love of animals and love of people. *Journal of Social Psychology, 116,* 299-300.

Rettig, K. D., Danes, S. M., & Bauer, J. W. (1989, November). *Family life quality: Theory, assessment, and replication.* Paper presented at the Preconference Workshop on Theory Construction and Research Methodology, National Council on Family Relations, New Orleans, LA.

Rogers, J., Hart, L. A., & Boltz, R. P. (1993). The role of pet dogs in casual conversations of elderly adults. *Journal of Social Psychology, 133,* 265-277.

Rowan, A. N., & Beck, A. M. (1994). The health benefits of human-animal interactions. *Anthrozoös, 7,* 85-89.

Russell, D., Peplau, L. A., & Cutrona, C. E. (1980). The Revised UCLA Loneliness Scale: Concurrent and discriminant validity evidence. *Journal of Personality and Social Psychology, 39,* 472-480.

Schutz, W. C. (1966). *The interpersonal underworld.* Palo Alto, CA: Science & Behavior Books.

Serpell, J. (1991). Beneficial effects of pet ownership on some aspects of human health and behavior. *Journal of the Royal Society of Medicine, 84,* 717-720.

Siegel, J. M. (1990). Stressful life events and use of physician services among the elderly: The moderating role of pet ownership. *Journal of Personality and Social Psychology, 58,* 1081-1086.

Spielberger, C. D., Gorsuch, R. L., & Lushene, R. E. (1970). *STAI manual for the State-Trait Anxiety Inventory ("Self-Evaluation Questionnaire").* Palo Alto, CA: Consulting Psychologists Press.

Stallones, L., Marx, M. B., Garrity, T. F., & Johnson, T. P. (1990). Pet ownership and attachment in relation to the health of U.S. adults, 21 to 64 years of age. *Anthrozoös, 4,* 100-112.

St. Yves, A., Freeston, M. H., Jacques, C., & Robitaille, C. (1990). Love of animals and interpersonal affectionate behavior. *Psychological Reports, 67,* 1067-1075.

Straede, C. M., & Gates, G. R. (1993). Psychological health in a population of Australian cat owners. *Anthrozoös, 6,* 30-42.

Templer, D., Salter, C., Dickey, S., Baldwin, R., & Veleber, D. (1981). The construction of a Pet Attitude Scale. *Psychological Record, 31,* 343-348.

Tucker, J. S., Friedman, H. S., Tsai, C. M., & Martin, L. R. (1995). Playing with pets and longevity among older people. *Psychology and Aging, 10,* 3-7.

Watson, N. L., & Weinstein, M. (1993). Pet ownership in relation to depression, anxiety, and anger in working women. *Anthrozoös, 6,* 135-138.

Wilson, C. C. (1991). The pet as an anxiolytic intervention. *Journal of Nervous and Mental Diseases, 179,* 482-489.

Zasloff, R. L., & Kidd, A. H. (1994). Loneliness and pet ownership among single women. *Psychological Reports, 75,* 747-752.

Perspectives on Animal-Assisted Activities and Therapy 2

Linda Hines
Maureen Fredrickson

Abstract

Animal-assisted activities and therapy (AAA/T), initially considered as worthwhile volunteer endeavors, are increasingly accepted as treatment options by the health care community. This chapter reviews reasons for the evolution of the roles of animals in health care facilities and other institutions. These reasons include popularization of studies on how animals affect human health and well-being, definition of the field of AAA/T, training of the animal handlers and health care professionals involved, evaluation and monitoring of therapy animals, development of varied service delivery programs, and documentation of the outcomes.

Popularization of Human-Animal Interaction Studies

Studies published in the 1980s demonstrated that contact with animals was healthy. These studies indicated that pets contributed to a child's development of nurturance and self-concept; promoted dialogue among family members, children, people with disabilities, and isolated

AUTHORS' NOTE: We thank Michelle Cobey, Resource Support Specialist at Delta Society, for her assistance in providing references for this article.

individuals; and contributed to physiological well-being, including survival of myocardial infarction, blood pressure reduction, and reduction in anxiety levels. Studies also demonstrated that pets mitigated the effects of bereavement in older persons and contributed to positive life satisfaction. These studies piqued the interest of the media, who introduced the findings to a wide audience in popular national magazines and a myriad of national and local newspapers. Print coverage was augmented by national and local television and radio interviews and feature stories. Scientific information summarized in lay language fed the growing public interest in anything to do with pets. Broad public awareness of these studies encouraged funding from the pet food industry and other sources for further studies. Responding to the growing literature, as well as increased public interest, the National Institutes of Health (NIH) convened a technology assessment workshop in September 1987, titled "Health Benefits of Pets." The working group drafted a report "to provide the scientific community with a synthesis of the current knowledge and a framework for future research, and to provide the public with the information it needs to make informed decisions regarding the health benefits of pets" (National Institutes of Health, 1988, p. 1).

Data from these scientific studies supported the experience of pet owners that animals can improve the quality of life for people. This inspired humane societies to encourage volunteers to visit residents of long-term care facilities with shelter puppies and kittens. Their goal was to share the benefits of interaction with pets with some of the loneliest people in society and, at the same time, to promote public good will for the organization and adoption of animals. Soon, dog clubs and other groups encouraged their members to establish such visits with pets. Initially referred to as "pet therapy," these informal programs brightened the days and brought laughter to people in countless nursing homes and other institutional settings. Early programs required little or no screening of animals or specific training for individuals accompanying the animals. Pet therapy was considered to be a pleasant diversionary program, and institutions welcomed a free activity as long as the program did not increase staff workload or pose significant risks to patient health and safety.

Concerns about patient safety, risk of zoonotic infection, risks to volunteers and animals, and lack of clearly documented benefits led health care professionals to demand criteria to establish and evaluate programs. Early programs were begun without documented processes or development of institutional policies or protocols for addressing these concerns and risks. Because of limited written materials on the early programs (Arkow, 1987; Hines, 1982; *People Pet Partnership Program,* 1993) each new program was left to reinvent the wheel. This slowed the implementation of new programs, as each institution struggled to define useful policy, identify risks, and determine effective procedures.

Definition of the Field

As the practice of bringing animals into health care facilities expanded in the 1980s, the term *pet therapy* became more of an impediment than an asset. First, licensed therapists argued that simply introducing animals into a setting did not meet definitions and criteria for therapy as understood in the health care professions and that volunteers did not qualify as therapists. Second, the plethora of terms used to describe these programs (*pet therapy, pet-assisted therapy, pet-facilitated psychotherapy*) led researchers and health care providers to conclude that there was lack of agreement as to the role of the animal and limited effectiveness from animal use (Blackshaw & Crowley, 1991; Draper, Gerber, & Layng, 1990; Noel de Tilly, 1991).

In the 1990s, the increased need for professionalism and credibility resulted in the development of the first comprehensive standards of practice. Now in its second edition, *Standards of Practice for Animal-Assisted Activities and Animal-Assisted Therapy* (Delta Society, 1996) defines the role of animals in therapeutic programs. Differentiation is made between programs that incorporate animals for purposes of entertainment or generalized population benefits, animal-assisted activities (AAA) and those that seek to cause a prescribed effect on specific patients, animal-assisted therapy (AAT). Definitions of these from the *Standards of Practice* follow.

> AAT is a goal-directed intervention in which an animal meeting specific criteria is an integral part of the treatment process. AAT is delivered and/or directed by a health or human service provider working within the scope of his/her profession. AAT is designed to promote improvement in human physical, social, emotional and/or cognitive functioning. AAT is provided in a variety of settings and may be group or individual in nature. The process is documented and evaluated. AAT is provided by a health or human service professional who includes an animal as part of his/her practice. Specific goals for each client have been identified by the professional, and progress is measured and recorded.

AAA provide opportunities for motivational, informational, and/or recreational benefits to enhance quality of life. AAA are delivered in a variety of environments by a specially trained professional, paraprofessional, and/or volunteer in association with animals that meet specific criteria. AAA activities involve animals visiting people. The same activity can be repeated with different people, unlike therapy that is tailored to a particular person or medical condition. (p. 50)

The *Standards of Practice* (Delta Society, 1996) also explores several areas of concern repeatedly identified by health care professionals and risk management personnel as central to decision-making processes. These areas include animal selection and husbandry (health and management), credentials and training of professional and voluntary personnel involved in AAA/T programs (continuing education, methodology, and performance evaluations), specific requirements for protocols and processes of operation (policies and procedures, organization and administration, and use management), and specific directions for recording data that may affect future programs (activity/treatment plans, infection control, and risk mitigation). As these standards are adopted, AAA/T has the potential to be recognized as a legitimate treatment choice that provides unique opportunities for professional growth. Incorporation of practice standards will encourage documentation of organizational, procedural, and reporting systems. Documentation of processes will highlight the similarities and differences in programs that can be evaluated and provide information regarding the therapeutic outcomes.

There is a tendency for some volunteers and uninformed health care providers to label any client-animal interaction as therapy from a concern that AAA have less value or importance or that AAA are not a serious component of resident/patient care; just the opposite is true. The majority of programs currently in existence are AAA programs that provide therapeutic benefits when undertaken by properly trained and screened people and animals (Delta Society, 1996). Anecdotal accounts of AAA programs describe a wide variety of benefits to clients, as well as staff, of recipient institutions. These benefits include increased empathy, outward focus, nurturing, rapport, entertainment, socialization, mental stimulation, physical contact/touch, relaxation, and sense of fulfillment.

Volunteers and institutional staff members have observed that the people in health care and educational settings experience benefits from animal contact that are similar to those recorded in early studies of human-animal interactions. Recent evaluations of AAA programs have begun to confirm the anecdotal evidence (Bernstein, Friedmann, & Malaspina, 1995; Fritz, Farver, Kass, & Hart, 1995; Holcomb & Meacham, 1989; Jessen, Cardiello, & Baun, 1996; Rosenkoetter, 1991). Such studies provide important credibility for informal, volunteer-initiated programs.

Many nursing homes and other long-term care facilities approve of AAA programs under the general supervision of an activity director. Volunteers bring in their own pets to visit clients. Commonly, there are no specific criteria regarding the duration of the visits or the process of the intervention. Volunteer-animal teams have been shown to produce measurable benefits in socialization between people, mental stimulation (e.g., memory recall), nurturing/outward focus, and entertainment.

Although programs meeting the definition of AAT are fewer in number and much more recent than AAA programs, they represent an area with great growth potential. More clinical studies are demonstrating quantifiable outcomes. Clearly documented intervention techniques are described in rehabilitation programs in which patient progress is easily quantifiable. Benefits to this population include improved fine motor skills, improved wheelchair skills, and improved standing balance (Allen & Blascovich, 1996; Bernard, 1995; Johnson, 1995; McLaughlin, 1996; Zapf, 1995). Although less quantifiable, psychosocial AAT goals include increased attention skills in adults with chronic mental illness and children diagnosed with attention deficit hyperactivity disorder, increased self-esteem, reduced anxiety during medical procedures, and increased social behaviors in abuse survivors (Bauman, Posner, Sachs, & Szita, 1991; Bernstein et al., 1995; Burch, 1992, 1995; Francis, 1991; Grunbaum, 1992; Katcher & Wilkins, 1994; Parker, 1996; Reichert, 1994; Woolverton, 1991).

Educational or cognitive goals have been less clearly measured or identified. A small number of studies of AAT interventions with children with learning disabilities and patients with Alzheimer's disease, however, show significantly increased vocabulary, increased long- or short-term memory, improved speech, and improved knowledge of concepts such as size and color (Baun, Batson, McCabe, & Wilson, 1995; Brockett, 1989; Bryant, 1995; A. Fristoe, personal interview, 1993; Hill, 1994; Katcher & Wilkins, 1995; Philippe, 1995; Ruth, 1992). Additional benefits of AAT interventions are frequently categorized as motivational and can include responses of willingness to be involved in a group activity, increased verbal interactions between group members, improved interactions with others, and increased interactions with staff (Bowes, 1991; Cawley, Cawley, & Retter, 1994; Kongable, 1990; Mallon, 1994; Prelewicz, 1993; Redefer & Goodman, 1989; Savishinsky, 1992).

Examples of AAT interventions that address specific goals include upper extremity exercise for stroke or head injury patients to increase strength, endurance, respiratory status, and independence in activities of daily living (Bernard, 1995) and the involvement of an animal as a contingent reinforcer to decrease tantrums and to teach a child to walk (Burch, 1995, 1996).

Training of Animal Handlers and Health Care Professionals

Animal Handler Volunteers

As the potential benefits to residents and patients from well-planned contacts with animals, and the potential liability from unplanned contacts, are realized, there is a demand from facility administrators for specialized training and screening procedures for both the people and animals. Three service delivery systems can provide trained volunteers: Volunteers can receive training independently, through a not-for-profit volunteer organization, or through a health care facility in-house volunteer training program.

The largest comprehensive training system for independent volunteers in the United States (and probably the world) is the Pet Partners Program®. Animal handler volunteers are trained at an all-day workshop by certified instructors or through a home study course, *Pet Partners Introductory Animal Handler's Skills Course* (1995). After successfully completing a written test, and after their animals complete health, aptitude, and skills testing, the volunteers are registered by Delta Society for 2 years. Continuing education is provided through a bimonthly newsletter and through seminars and workshops at Delta annual conferences. Registered volunteers are covered by liability insurance. Reregistration depends on successful service in an AAA or AAT program and participation in continuing education.

The Pet Partners course includes units identified in the *Standards of Practice* (Delta Society, 1996) that should be part of any volunteer education program. They are

- Animal handlers (needs and responsibilities)
- Animals (health and skills/aptitude requirements, protecting the animal)
- Clients (interaction techniques)
- Visiting (general techniques)
- Facilities (regulations and policies, staff relationships, reducing risk)

Health Care Professionals

For AAA/T programs to truly benefit clients, it is essential that the staff of health care facilities also receive training. Without specialized training in the ways animal contact affects clients, and potential contraindications, therapists may incorporate inappropriate animals and jeopardize safety or may not maximize treatment options. Activity directors, who often oversee AAA, must have realistic expectations for visiting teams. They must ensure the development and implementation of protocols to protect the facility and its residents. Independently managed volunteer programs work with the facilities in which their volunteers serve to provide such orientation to staff and to assist in developing policies and procedures.

Nurses, physical and occupational therapists, psychiatrists, and other health care professionals require methodology-based training on techniques of AAT. This is difficult to obtain in any consistent manner. Educational and experiential guidelines are being developed to address these concerns, setting the stage for acceptance of AAA/T within the health care field, a process that still is in its beginning stages. Seminars and workshops at national and international professional meetings provide one means for learning techniques and protocols. In-service training provides another avenue of learning for health care professionals.

Evaluating and Monitoring Animals

In the 1970s and 1980s, many visiting pet programs encouraged volunteers to work with shelter animals. By the 1990s, however, all major humane associations and veterinary organizations in the United States recommended against such a practice. Visiting strange settings with unpredictable people and unusual noises stresses the animals, especially young animals that are awaiting adoption ("Shelter Animals," 1992). Animals with unknown health histories and unknown behavior patterns are put in contact with vulnerable people, increasing the risk of zoonotic infection or injury. Also, this practice may reduce the effectiveness of the interaction because well-trained animals can have skills that enhance interactions with others. In addition, the return of the same animal through time aids in establishing a relationship with clients or patients (New, 1995). In AAT programs, this relationship is often the goal of treatment.

Concerns about zoonotic infections and public health and environmental issues involving animals in treatment are the most frequently stated reasons for not incorporating AAA/T programs. Curiously, these concerns have never been substantiated. Epidemiologic studies are frequently cited as sources of facts regarding zoonotic risk of animal contact. Yet an informal review of zoonotic illnesses reported to the Centers for Disease Control (S. Duncan, personal communication, 1996) revealed no reported incidents in institutions hosting AAA/T programs. A handful of studies indicate that properly cared-for animals do not pose additional health risks and that the benefits outweigh the small, easily preventable risks involved (Anderson, Reid, & Jennings, 1992; Kale, 1992; "Patients' Best Friend," 1992; Waltner-Toews & Ellis, 1994).

Practitioners in the field recognize the importance of involving only carefully selected visiting and resident animals. As explained in the *Standards of Practice* (Delta Society, 1996), "Animals that participate in AAA/T are purposefully selected, healthy, safe, and meet risk management criteria. They possess appropriate aptitude, are an appropriate size and age, and demonstrate appropriate skills for their participation to be beneficial to all team members" (pp. 41-42).

The Delta Society Task Force on Animal Screening developed minimum screening protocols for animals involved in AAA/T. From a survey of more than 600 evaluators for various programs, the Pet Partners Aptitude Test® (PPAT) (1993) was created, which evaluates the animal-handler team as a working unit. The task force recommended that animal-handler teams be reevaluated every 2 years to account for changes in aptitude due to health, aging, and life events. In addition, it identified a second critical factor in successful screening of animals: the evaluator's knowledge of AAA/T. Unlike show-ring competition or trips to the park, the AAA/T setting presents unique situations and challenges to the animal and handler. Each client population responds differently to animals, based on behavioral, physical, and environmental dynamics. The Pet Partners Program

requires 12 contact hours of training and completion of written and prac-
ticum tests for final certification of animal evaluators.

Most animals involved in AAA/T visit a facility along with the handler,
who may be a volunteer or a staff person at the facility. Some animals are
selected and placed as permanent residents of a facility. Serious concerns
have arisen about placement of resident animals. The idea that by simply
being in an institution the animal is therapeutic is erroneous. Animals
placed without thorough planning, selection, and staff commitment can be
improperly cared for and even injured. Behavioral problems resulting from
poor training or boredom reduce effectiveness in stimulating residents or
cause fear or injury. If a facility makes a commitment of resources and
trained staff, resident animals can be a successful model (Lee, Zeglan,
Ryan, Gowing, & Hines, 1987; Thomas, 1994).

Development of Service Delivery Programs

Three primary models exist for the delivery of AAA/T. In the first
model, individuals—whether volunteers or therapists—work independently with one or more institutions. In the second model, an organized
group recruits, trains, and monitors volunteers and schedules their interactions in various facilities. In the third model, a facility such as a hospital
or nursing home recruits, trains, and monitors its own corps of volunteers
and schedules their interactions with the facility's patients or residents.

Independent Animal Handlers/Therapists

Individual Delta Society Pet Partners attend an animal handler skills
workshop or order a home study course and training videotape to receive
training. They contact the Delta Society office for the name of a Delta-
certified animal evaluator to screen their pets. Then the individual contacts
a nearby facility and arranges to visit residents or patients.

Organized Group That Visits Facilities

National Capital Therapy Dogs, Inc. (NCTD), a not-for-profit organization located in Baltimore, Maryland, provides visiting animal-people

teams to a variety of settings in the greater Washington, D.C., area. NCTD recruits, trains, and schedules volunteers for all sites. Volunteers are provided classroom and on-site training through a mentor system. Dogs are screened by NCTD members designated for this task. Volunteers and their animals attend regular meetings and training sessions.

This model has enabled NCTD to provide services in institutions with extremely fragile populations, such as NIH pediatric AIDS and oncology units. Board members meet with key staff of each facility and institute specific policies and procedures for each site. The one-to-one contact with facility administration and risk management personnel has enabled NCTD volunteers to develop and work within stringent screening and behavioral criteria, resulting in an opportunity to bring AAA and AAT to populations formerly considered too fragile medically to receive visits. Visits are free to the institution because NCTD pays for expenses of training, screening, and volunteer management through donations.

Another example of an independent organization providing AAA/T services is Hope Therapy, Galveston, Texas. This organization is a not-for-profit health care facility specializing in rehabilitation therapies. A large percentage of services are provided through the therapeutic horseback riding program. Hope Therapy also provides services in local facilities. Facilities are charged a fee for services; AAT services are billed as indicated by the directing professional occupational therapist, physiotherapist, and so on. People involved in the Hope Therapy program are employees of Hope Therapy and are paid and trained in AAA/T by that organization. As with NCTD, direct contact with administration and risk management personnel has resulted in visits to medically fragile individuals.

Organized Volunteers Within a Facility

Denver Children's Hospital operates one of the oldest AAA programs in the United States. Volunteers are trained and their animals screened and medically evaluated through the hospital volunteer auxiliary. The auxiliary has organized local veterinarians and experienced volunteers to provide animal screening. Because the hospital demands extensive medical screening for animals involved in the program, veterinarians take samples for no fee and the hospital runs cultures at no cost. A volunteer coordinator on the staff of the hospital schedules all visits and tracks animal and volunteer renewal. Volunteers are approved to work only in Denver Children's Hospital because they are insured through the hospital volunteer program. Clients are referred to the services by physicians. No fees are charged to clients for the service.

A second example of a facility-managed program can be found at Tyler Rehabilitation Hospital in Tyler, Texas. The program is part of the rehabilitation service, and a staff occupational therapist manages the program. AAT services are provided as part of patient rehabilitation goals and billed as traditional occupational therapy, physiotherapy, or speech therapy services. Volunteers work with patients at the direction of the health care professional. Volunteers receive training, and their animals are screened by the OT in charge of the program. AAA visits are provided to all patients in the facility on a regular basis.

As with the Denver program, volunteers have been limited to working only at Tyler because insurance is linked to the facility. To expand their volunteers' experiences and opportunities, Tyler Rehabilitation Hospital now trains and registers volunteers through the Pet Partners Program. A large number of facility-based programs, as well as organized groups that visit a number of local facilities, offer their volunteers registration with the Pet Partners Program. This provides volunteers with transportable insurance, continuing education, and a link to people with similar interests and goals nationwide.

Evaluation and Documentation

Many questions still exist regarding the effects of AAA/T in various health care settings. Although written almost 10 years ago, advice from the NIH Technology Assessment Workshop is still relevant.

> Methodologies for future research can begin without explicit hypothesis and proceed from descriptive studies of representative and, hopefully, random samples. There is nothing intrinsically wrong with extrapolating from attitudinal information as long as the sample is representative of the target population. It should be remembered that samples of convenience are prone to bias, and interpretation must be limited and made with great care. If the hypothesis is supported, research could proceed to cross-sectional and retrospective studies and then to long-range prospective investigations. A causal association between animal contact and human health can be demonstrated only by prospective studies. (National Institutes of Health, 1988, p. 5).

The greatest barriers to the development of sound scientific studies have been poor definitions of AAA/T goals, lack of agreement on means of measurement and documentation, and use of small sample sizes (Voelker, 1995). The health care industry bases treatment decisions on outcome data demonstrating that the intervention results in progress toward or meeting the identified goal. It has been difficult to show that AAA/T interventions alone produced the desired results. Several studies that compared results between animal-assisted interventions and puppet or volunteer interventions indicated no differences in the benefits (Bumsted, 1988; Hendy, 1987; Nielsen & Delude, 1994; Tipton, 1994; Vaughan, 1990). Little attention has been given to those studies that indicate limited or no benefits are found (Chinner & Dalziel, 1991; Struckus, 1989; Taylor, 1993).

Much remains to be learned about the ways animals can be incorporated as a health care option. Studies of the long-term effects of animal-assisted interventions are needed (Wilson & Netting, 1987). Programs that incorporate animals in milieu treatment report exciting results, including reduced staff turnover, reduced prescription for psychotropic medication, reduced violence, and lowered death rate (Haynes, 1991; Lee, 1983; Thomas, 1994). Reproducible long-term effects can change the focus of treatment in the years to come.

The final analysis of this form of complementary therapy must include information on the process, as well as outcomes, of AAA/T. Careful documentation of how institutional attitudes and policies change when animals are allowed in the facility may provide valuable insights into the success of these programs. It is possible that the introduction of animals into institutional settings results in significant changes in the perceptions of the staff regarding the patient's abilities, progress, or improvement (Burch, 1996; Cole & Gawlinski, 1995). Frequently, the most valuable aspect of AAA/T programs is that they enable caregivers to believe that the patient has similarities to themselves and capabilities beyond initial impressions.

Next Steps

Establishment of certification for practitioners of AAA/T is an important next step to increase professionalism in this field. The existence of professional credentials, continuing education requirements, and peer review will provide practitioners with guidelines for quality practice.

It will serve to reduce the confusion of services offered and assure the health care community of measurable standards of practice for those providing services.

Development of advanced continuing education materials for health care professionals and volunteers is another essential step. Currently, educational programs focus on entry-level personnel and do not address the needs of those with moderate experience. A goal of the Delta Society Task Force on AAA/T curriculum is to develop AAA/T training to the extent that it becomes a recognized speciality within nursing, occupational and physical therapy, special education, and other areas.

One of the greatest challenges in the field is convincing health care professionals to adopt standards, use standardized terminology, and require training of volunteers/staff and screening and retesting of animals involved in programs. Such procedures must become routine and not exceptions if the field is to gain respect and grow. Adoption of these procedures will also aid in changing public policy whereby animals are excluded by law from acute care facilities.

Animal screening protocols must be tested for validity and continually improved. Retrospective analysis of incident reports and pass/fail rates could lead to an understanding of the behavioral and training requirements for safe and reliable animals. At this time, the greatest attention has been directed toward screening dogs. In many facilities, dogs may be less effective than other species of animals. Screening for these animals, especially nondomestic animals, is still in its infancy.

As previously stated, data regarding the risks of transmission of zoonotic disease in AAA/T programs are minimal. This may be because of self-monitoring by the facilities and personnel involved. With the incorporation of animals in health care facilities growing, however, it will be important to monitor this aspect. As animals visit more medically fragile people, the risk of infection and injury grows. At the same time, exposing animals to resistant forms of human disease such as tuberculosis and some forms of staphylococcus could pose a risk to the animals. By working closely with veterinarians and public health specialists, practitioners can ensure the safety of both the people and the animals in these programs.

Medical interest in the benefits of human-animal interactions continues to be a major barrier to growth in the field of AAA/T. Although the pet industry promotes the health benefits of contacts with animals, this interest has not spread to the health care industry. It is reported that many academics treat those who participate in studies of human-animal interactions with amused tolerance (Allen & Blascovich, 1996; Rowan, 1995). Even in the area of cardiac health, in which studies have clearly indicated pet ownership as a positive factor, the medical community does not routinely incorporate this information into patient care.

Most AAA/T research to date does not study people who are ill or in institutions. This must change if the field is to gain the data it needs to develop techniques, identify patient populations who can benefit, and create educational materials for health care professionals. Practitioners can begin to build this database by completing well-written case studies. As Rowan (1995) stated, "What the well-turned anecdote can do for politics, . . . a detailed case study can also do to stimulate the interest of the medical and public health professions" (p. 131).

In a recent article Voelker (1995) describes positive patient interactions in a few AAT programs and provides photographs of the children and adults helped. Then Voelker states the current attitude of the medical community and shows the path ahead: "The biggest challenge facing advocates who say animal-assisted therapy improves outcomes can be summed up in two words: Prove it" (p. 1898).

References

Allen, K., & Blascovich, J. (1996). The value of service dogs for people with severe ambulatory disabilities. *Journal of the American Medical Association,, 275*(13), 1001-1006.

Anderson, W. P., Reid, C. M., & Jennings, G. L. (1992). Pet ownership and risk factors for cardiovascular disease. *Medical Journal of Australia, 157,* 298-301.

Arkow, P. (1987). *"Pet therapy": A study and resource guide for the use of companion animals in selected therapies* (5th ed.). Colorado Springs, CO: Humane Society of the Pikes Peak Region.

Bauman, L., Posner, M., Sachs, K., & Szita, R. (1991). The effects of animal-assisted therapy on communication patterns with chronic schizophrenics. *Latham Letter, 13*(4), 3-5, 17-19.

Baun, M. M., Batson, K., McCabe, B. W., & Wilson, C. M. (1995, September). *The effect of a therapy dog on socialization and physiologic indicators of stress in persons diagnosed with Alzheimer's disease.* Paper presented at the Seventh International Conference on Human-Animal Interactions: Animals, Health, and Quality of Life, Geneva, Switzerland.

Bernstein, P., Friedmann, E., & Malaspina, A. (1995). Pet programs can provide a novel source of interaction in long-term facilities. In A. L. Ptak, Studies of loneliness: Recent research into the effects of companion animals on lonely people. *InterActions, 13*(1), 7.

Bernard, S. (1995). *Animal assisted therapy: A guide for health care professionals and volunteers.* Whitehouse, TX: Therapet L. L. C.

Blackshaw, J. K., & Crowley, P. (1991). A survey to determine the presence and claimed therapeutic use of pets in selected institutions. *Australian Veterinary Practitioner, 21*(1), 11-13.

Bowes, L. G. (1991). *Pet assisted therapy at an Edmonton auxiliary hospital.* Unpublished master's thesis, University of Alberta, Edmonton, Alberta, Canada.

Brockett, S. (1989, November). *A classroom canine companion curriculum.* Paper presented at 8th annual conference of the Delta Society, Parsippany, NJ.

Bryant, B. K. (1995, September). *Animal assisted therapy within the context of daily institutional life.* Paper presented at the Seventh International Conference on Human-Animal Interactions: Animals, Health, and Quality of Life, Geneva, Switzerland.

Bumsted, D. L. (1988). *The effect of pet therapy on the self-care of the elderly.* Unpublished master's thesis, Southern Connecticut State University, New Haven.

Burch, M. R. (1992). Behavior treatment of drug exposed children. *Children Today, 21*(1), 12-15.

Burch, M. R. (1995). The role of pets in therapeutic programmes: Animal-assisted therapy. In I. Robinson (Ed.), *The Waltham book of human-animal interaction: Benefits and responsibilities of pet ownership* (pp. 57-60). Oxford, UK: Pergamon/Kidlington.

Burch, M. R. (1996). *Volunteering with your pet: How to get involved in animal-assisted therapy with any kind of pet.* New York: Howell.

Cawley, R., Cawley, D., & Retter, K. (1994). Therapeutic horseback riding and self-concept in adolescents with special educational needs. *Anthrozoös, 7*(2), 129-134.

Chinner, T. L., & Dalziel, F. R. (1991). An exploratory study on the viability and efficacy on a pet-facilitated therapy project within a hospice. *Journal of Palliative Care, 7*(4), 13-20.

Cole, K. M., & Gawlinski, A. (1995). Animal-assisted therapy in the intensive care unit: A staff nurse's dream comes true. *Nursing Clinics of North America, 30*(3), 529-537.

Delta Society 2nd ed. (1996). *Standards of practice for animal-assisted activities and animal-assisted therapy.* Renton, WA: Author.

Draper, R. J., Gerber, G., & Layng, M. (1990). Defining the role of pet animals in psychotherapy. *Psychiatric Journal of the University of Ottawa, 15*(3), 169-172.

Francis, G. M. (1991). Here come the puppies: The power of the human-animal bond. *Holistic Nursing Practice, 5*(2), 38-41.

Fritz, C. L., Farver, T. B., Kass, P. H., & Hart, L. A. (1995). Association with companion animals and the expression of noncognitive symptoms in Alzheimer's patients. *Journal of Nervous and Mental Disease, 183*(7), 459-463.

Grunbaum, L. (1992). *The effect of animal-assisted therapy on anxiety in acutely ill patients.* Unpublished master's thesis, San Francisco State University, San Francisco.

Haynes, M. (1991). Pet therapy: Program lifts spirits, reduces violence in institution's mental health unit. *Corrections Today, 53*(5), 120-122.

Hendy, H. M. (1987). Effects of pet and/or people visits on nursing home residents. *International Journal of Aging and Human Development, 25*(4), 279-291.

Hill, C. (1994, October). *Curriculum based animal assisted activities.* Paper presented at the 13th annual conference of the Delta Society: Pets, People, and the Natural World, New York.

Hines, L. M. (1982). Establishing a people-pet partnership program. [Brochure]. Alameda, CA: Latham Foundation.

Holcomb, R., & Meacham, R. (1989). Effectiveness of an animal-assisted therapy program in an inpatient psychiatric unit. *Anthrozoös, 2*(4), 259-273.

Jessen, J., Cardiello, F., & Baun, M. M. (1996). Avian companionship in alleviation of depression, loneliness and low morale of older adults in skilled rehabilitation units. *Psychological Reports, 78,* 339-348.

Johnson, K. A. (1995). [Pet-assisted therapy program]. Letter stating results of program at Shriners Hospitals for Crippled Children, Chicago Unit.

Kale, M. (1992). Kids & animals: A comforting hospital combination. *InterActions, 10*(3), 17-21.

Katcher, A., & Wilkins, G. G. (1994). Helping children with attention-deficit hyperactive and conduct disorders through animal-assisted therapy and education. *InterActions, 12*(4), 5-9.

Katcher, A., & Wilkins, G. G. (1995, September). *Evaluation of an animal-assisted therapy program by comparison of success in programs with behavioral outcomes in other contexts.* Paper presented at the 7th International Conference on Human-Animal Interactions: Animals, Health, and Quality of Life, Geneva, Switzerland.

Kongable, L. G. (1990). Pet therapy for Alzheimer's patients: A survey. *Journal of Long-Term Care Administration, 13*(3), 17-21.

Lee, D. R. (1983, May). Pet therapy helping patients through troubled times. *California Veterinarian,* 24-25, 40.

Lee, R. L., Zeglan, M. E., Ryan, T., Gowing, C. B., & Hines, L. M. (1987). *Guidelines: Animals in nursing homes* (Rev. ed.). Renton, WA: Delta Society and California Veterinary Medical Association.

Mallon, G. P. (1994). Cow as co-therapist: Utilization of farm animals as therapeutic aides with children in residential treatment. *Child & Adolescent Social Work Journal, 11*(6), 455-474.

McLaughlin, C. (1996). Bow-wow: What a difference animal assistance can make. *Advance for Physical Therapists, 7*(4), 10-11.

National Institutes of Health. (1988). *Summary of working group on health benefits of pets* (DHHS Publication No. 216-107). Washington, DC: Government Printing Office.

Nielsen, J. A., & Delude, L. A. (1994). Pets as adjunct therapists in a residence for former psychiatric patients. *Anthrozoös, 7*(3), 166-171.

New, J. C. (1995, September). *Quality of life of companion animals.* Paper presented at the Seventh International Conference on Human-Animal Interactions: Animals, Health, and Quality of Life, Geneva, Switzerland.

Noel de Tilly, J. (1991). Animals and therapy. *Veterinary Technician, 12*(6), 455-459.

Parker, H. (1996). JAMA asks animal-assisted therapy to prove it: News and analysis. *Anthrozoös, 8*(4), 244-245.

Patients' best friend? Hospital dogs raise spirits, not infection rates. (1992, December). *Hospital Infection Control,* 162-164.

People Pet Partnership Program. (1993). Pullman, WA: People Pet Partnership Program.

Pet Partners Aptitude Test. (n.d.). Renton, WA: Delta Society.

Pet Partners introductory animal handler skills course. (1995). Renton, WA: Delta Society.

Philippe, S. (1995). *Animal-assisted therapy (educational and psychological aspects) with dogs for psychotic and autistic children.* Paper presented at the 7th International Conference on Human-Animal Interactions: Animals, Health, and Quality of Life, Geneva, Switzerland.

Prelewicz, T. N. (1993). *The effects of animal-assisted therapy on loneliness in elderly residents of a long-term care facility utilizing Roy's adaptation model.* Unpublished master's thesis, D'Youville College, Buffalo, NY.

Redefer, L. A., & Goodman, J. F. (1989). Brief report: Pet-facilitated therapy with autistic children. *Journal of Autism and Developmental Disorders, 19*(3), 461-467.

Reichert, E. (1994). Play and animal-assisted therapy: A group-treatment model for sexually abused girls ages 9-13. *Family Therapy, 21*(1), 55-62.

Rosenkoetter, M. (1991). Health promotion: The influence of pets on life patterns in the home. *Holistic Nursing Practice, 5*(2), 42-51.

Rowan, A. N. (1995). Medical disinterest in human-animal bond research? *Anthrozoös, 8*(3), 130-131.

Ruth, R. (1992). Animals are helping children overcome physical and emotional challenges. *InterActions, 10*(1), 16-18.

Savishinsky, J. S. (1992). Intimacy, domesticity and pet therapy with the elderly: Expectation and experience among nursing home volunteers. *Social Science and Medicine, 34*(12), 1325-1334.

Shelter animals inappropriate for visiting program. (1992). *Pet Partners Newsletter, 2*(6).

Struckus, J. E. (1989). *The use of pet-facilitated therapy in the treatment of depression in the elderly: A behavioral conceptualization of treatment effect.* Unpublished master's thesis, University of Massachusetts, Worcester.

Taylor, E. (1993). Effects of animals on eye contact and vocalizations of elderly residents in a long term care facility. *Physical and Occupational Therapy in Geriatrics, 11*(4), 61-71.

Thomas, W. H. (1994). *The Eden alternative: Nature, hope and nursing homes.* Columbia: University of Missouri.

Tipton, J. L. (1994). *Pet therapy for multiply handicapped, technology dependent children.* Unpublished master's thesis, East Carolina University, Greenville, NC.

Vaughan, B. K. (1990). *Pet and patient: Enhancing nursing home life.* Unpublished master's thesis, California State University, Long Beach.

Voelker, R. (1995). Puppy love can be therapeutic, too. *Journal of the American Medical Association, 274*(24), 1897-1899.

Waltner-Toews, D., & Ellis, A. (1994). *Good for your animals, good for you: How to live and work with animals in activity and therapy programs and stay healthy.* Guelph, Ontario, Canada: University of Guelph.

Wilson, C. C., & Netting, F. E. (1987). New directions: Challenges for human-animal bond research and the elderly. *Journal of Applied Gerontology, 6,* 189-200.

Woolverton, M. C. (1991, October). *Reducing children's stress during physical examination by having them play with animals during the procedure.* Paper presented at the 10th annual conference of the Delta Society, Portland, OR.

Zapf, S. S. (1995). *Functional independence in occupational performance areas and psychosocial components in individuals with spinal cord injury who use assistance dogs.* Unpublished master's thesis, Texas Woman's University, Denton.

Hippotherapy and Therapeutic Riding 3

An International Review

Jane Copeland Fitzpatrick
Jean M. Tebay

Abstract

A horse, a therapist, a horse expert, and a person with a movement problem present the potential for hippotherapy—a medical treatment for people of all ages with movement dysfunction. Hippotherapy, one aspect of the broader field of therapeutic riding, employs the rhythmic, dynamic movement of the horse to influence the client's posture, balance, and mobility without having the client attempt to control the horse. Results from a survey of the member nations of the Federation of Riding for the Disabled showed that the practice of hippotherapy has expanded worldwide. The primary professional practitioners of hippotherapy are physical therapists with advanced training; other health professionals such as occupational therapists, speech therapists, and psychologists are also receiving training in hippotherapy. Research documenting hippotherapy as a treatment for neurologically involved clients is currently being conducted by individuals in several nations. Published studies can be found in the proceedings of international congresses on therapeutic riding and in scientific journals.

Introduction to Therapeutic Riding

❧ It has been nearly 50 years since Mme. Lis Hartel, a courageous woman with poliomyelitis and a severe walking impairment, made astounding history by winning a silver medal at the 1952 Olympic Games in Helsinki, Finland. Her success gave impetus to the embryonic concept of using the horse to help rehabilitate—both medically and psychologically—people with disabilities (Davies, 1988).

Since that time, a large field of endeavor has developed to improve the quality of life of individuals with disabilities through the use of equine-related activities (C. Klüwer, 1992, 1994). In the last half century, the unique healing qualities that the horse has for human bodies and minds have been recognized. As a result, the term *therapeutic riding* is used to describe all the rehabilitative uses of the horse (Engel, 1992, 1994; North American Riding for the Handicapped Association, 1993).

As therapeutic riding has grown and diversified worldwide, terminology to describe the different ways the horse is used for people with disabilities has evolved. Nearly all the organizations that offer equine-related activities for persons who are disabled provide riding for the disabled (Riding for the Disabled Association, 1984). In this activity, the recreation or sport of horseback riding and driving is adapted to specifically fit the needs of each participant. This could include the use of special reins, stirrups, or a specially designed saddle (Armstrong-Esther, Sandilands, Myco, & Miller, 1988; Britton, 1991; Joswick, Kittredge, McCowan, McParland, & Woods, 1986; Rosenzweig, 1987).

In *equine-assisted psychotherapy,* horse activities (e.g., riding and vaulting) are specifically designed to coordinate with the overall psychotherapeutic treatment of the patient (B. Klüwer, 1994; C. Klüwer, 1988; Scheidhacker, 1994a). Goals often are ego strengthening, self-confidence, and social competence. Scheidhacker (1994b) states that "horse riding is a therapy full of pleasure, where deep emotions can be experienced. The feeling . . . of being able to perceive oneself and of being able to establish a relation with one's surroundings is essential for a way out of the psychic illness" (p. 99). Another application of therapeutic riding for a patient with anorexia nervosa has been described by Leimer (1993).

The horse has also been used to design and implement educational goals for school-age children with learning problems. This use of the horse is referred to as *remedial educational riding and vaulting* (Heipertz, Heipertz, Kröger, & Kuprian, 1981; Kröger, 1992). At the British Fortune Center, a special type of riding education called Further Education Through Horse Mastership educates students who have left traditional educational settings (Baillie, 1985). In this setting, the horse is used as a strong motivator for accomplishing precisely designed educational goals. In cases in which behavior is a component of the overall student problem, the riding or vaulting program can also include behavioral goals (Cawley, Cawley, & Retter, 1993).

The common thread in riding for the disabled, equine-assisted psychotherapy, and remedial educational riding and vaulting is that the horse is used to improve the quality of life of individuals with disabilities. The individual learns the skills necessary to ride, vault, or drive. In another therapeutic use of the horse, the medical use, the rider—now called a client or patient—*does not* attempt to learn riding skills. This medical use of the horse is called *hippotherapy* and is based on the transfer of movement from the horse to the client (Baker, 1994; Cohen, 1992; Copeland, 1992; Heipertz et al., 1981; Strauss, 1991).

As therapeutic riding gained in popularity during the 1960s, this unique medical use of the horse, hippotherapy, was drawing increased attention from the medical community. Therapists in several countries began to define and describe the treatment technique of hippotherapy, explaining its use with a clientele having neurological and orthopedic symptoms to improve posture, mobility, and balance.

Hippotherapy

To obtain a better understanding of the medical use of the horse, a survey of the member nations of the Federation of Riding for the Disabled International was conducted. Twenty-three responses were obtained from 21 countries; multiple responses were obtained from one country. The variance in responses, however, was so great from the same member country that each was included as a separate entity. As a means of minimizing definitional problems, two definitions of hippotherapy used in curricula taught by the American Hippotherapy Association (AHA) were presented in the survey (i.e., classic hippotherapy and a somewhat broader definition of hippotherapy that includes a reference to sensory processing).

According to the AHA (1995),

> Hippotherapy (i.e., treatment with the help of the horse) comes from the Greek word *hippos,* meaning horse. Specially trained physical and occupational therapists use this medical treatment for clients with movement dysfunction. In classic hippotherapy, the horse influences the client, rather than the client controlling the horse. The client is positioned on, and actively responds to the movement of, the therapy horse. The therapist directs the movement of the horse, analyzes the client's responses, and adjusts the treatment accordingly. The goals of classic hippotherapy are to improve the client's posture, balance, mobility, and function. (p. 12)

The second definition adopted by the AHA (1995) is a functional definition used in its introductory curriculum. This definition states how the treatment approach is currently being implemented in the United States and Canada. More specifically, functional hippotherapy

> is a treatment approach that uses the movement of the horse on the basis of principles of classic hippotherapy, neuromotor function and sensory processing. It is a treatment that uses activities on the horse that are meaningful to the client. It provides a controlled environment and graded sensory input designed to elicit appropriate adaptive responses from the client. It does not teach specific skills, but rather provides a foundation of improved neuromotor function and sensory processing that can be generalized to a wide range of activities outside of treatment. Hippotherapy is used primarily to achieve physical goals but may also effect psychological, cognitive, behavioral and communication outcomes. Hippotherapy is used by licensed health professionals having a strong background in posture and movement, neuromotor function, and sensory processing. (p. 13)

Survey respondents were asked if they agreed or disagreed in principle with these definitions. Twenty-three responses representing 21 countries were received. The classic hippotherapy definition was endorsed by 17 respondents representing 16 countries as conceptually correct. The respondents from Germany, Switzerland, and the Netherlands indicated agreement in principle with the classic hippotherapy definition, with minor changes. Other countries surveyed, including Australia, Austria, Belgium, England, Hong Kong, Ireland, Israel, Italy, Luxembourg, New Zealand, Portugal, and Singapore also use hippotherapy in the classic manner.

Two countries responded that the functional definition refers to a treatment approach other than hippotherapy. In Finland, the term *riding therapy* replaces *functional hippotherapy;* in Germany, *therapeutic riding* or *rehabilitation riding* is used.

The Swiss Group for Hippotherapy refers to its treatment approach as Hippotherapy-K, a trademark treatment based on the work of physiotherapist Ursula Künzle (1995) and performed with clients who are neurologically impaired. Künzle's survey response defined Hippotherapy-K as this:

> The movement of the *small* horse's walk is used as a therapeutic medium in neurological rehabilitation. It needs a medical prescription and is carried out by physiotherapists with special postgraduate training. The therapists help obtain the optimal transfer of the movement from the horse to the patient. In Hippotherapy-K, riding is not the goal; the patient does not have any active influence on the horse. The goals are relaxation of the pelvic region, promotion of postural reactions, and promotion and preservation of balance in the sitting position.

The Deutsche Gruppe für Hippotherapie, one of three respondents from Germany, embraces the concepts of Hippotherapy-K and uses a similar definition, stressing that hippotherapy is a medical/therapeutic treatment in neurology that uses the movements of the walking horse as a therapeutic medium. The treatment goals include improvement of circulation and improvement of selective movements between parts of the body (trunk), as well as the improvement of posture, balance, and mobility.

Austrian physiotherapist Emmy Tauffkirchen (1992) defines hippotherapy as a "physiotherapeutical treatment based on neurophysiological principles. This includes using the help of the horse to treat neuromotor functions as well as sensory, psychological and cognitive abilities" (p. 124). Therapists in Belgium, Brazil, Finland, and France have expanded the base of classic hippotherapy to emphasize psychological aspects of disability, resulting in a more holistic approach. American and Canadian therapists have also broadened the classic definition of hippotherapy to include more emphasis on sensory processing. In Belgium, speech therapy is an important part of hippotherapy. Therapists in Australia, Hong Kong, New Zealand, and Singapore have only recently started offering hippotherapy, and all endorsed the survey definitions. Norway indicated that therapists have not yet adopted a specific definition.

Terminology varies from one country to another. Some countries, such as Spain, refer to all therapeutic uses of the horse as hippotherapy. Adding to the confusion, media reports often refer to all therapeutic riding as hippotherapy. The use of the medical treatment term *hippotherapy* to refer to all types of therapeutic riding negates the specialty and makes it difficult for therapists to bill those treatments that are physician-prescribed medical applications of the movement of the horse.

Another problem encountered when defining hippotherapy relates to its relative newness and to the nature of all therapeutic interventions. Therapies and therapeutic techniques evolve as new information and research become available. There is always a need to delineate new therapeutic techniques and theories, and each delineation necessitates slight variations and changes in terminology. That the term *hippotherapy* has survived for more than 30 years and is generally understood by physiotherapists in 20 countries indicates its general acceptance and viability. Once a professional community can agree on what constitutes a therapeutic treatment for a patient's condition, then this concept can be communicated to the general public, the media, and the institutions responsible for paying for the service.

As defined by all 23 respondents, hippotherapy has many observable similarities. All survey respondents agreed that a typical hippotherapy treatment session consists of these elements:

- A client with movement dysfunction usually resulting from neurological impairment
- A horse moving on at the walk
- A physician's written referral for the client
- A physiotherapist with specialized training who analyzes the client's movement prior to and during the hippotherapy treatment, making adjustments to ensure the optimal transfer of the movement of the horse's back to the client
- A client in a sitting position on the horse
- A client responding to but not influencing the horse's movement
- A horse handler who controls the horse according to the therapist's directions

In addition to these basic attributes, most countries surveyed have additional characteristics that describe hippotherapy in their locale (Cirillo, 1994; Strauss, 1991). These involve educational requirements and training programs for therapists, types of clients, types of horses, horse equipment, training and handling techniques employed, and methods of payment for treatment.

Training

☙ Hippotherapy requires advanced training of the therapist. In countries in which hippotherapy has been practiced for longer periods, formalized educational programs leading to certification or licensure exist (Brown & Tebay, 1994; La Thérapie, 1995; Riede, 1986, 1988; Strauss, 1993; Tebay, Rowley, Copeland, & Glasow, 1988). Austria, Germany, and Switzerland offer courses to physiotherapists that are given in two or three sections with an opportunity to study and practice between sessions. Of the survey respondents, 12 countries offer specialized training in hippo- therapy for physiotherapists (Australia, Austria, Belgium, Brazil, Canada, England, France, Finland, Germany, Israel, Switzerland, and the United States). Several of the surveyed countries include occupational therapists in their advanced training courses. Brazil includes psychologists and requires their presence at hippotherapy sessions. At the time of the survey, Finland reported having trained approximately 50 riding therapists, including physiotherapists, occupational therapists, special teachers for persons who are disabled, psychologists, and psychiatrists. In Finland, individuals who provide hippotherapy and/or *heilpädagogisches reiten* receive the same 2-year training given in three sessions. Luxembourg requires advanced training but did not state how or where it was given.

Austria, France, Germany, and Switzerland offer certification, licensure, or some standardized method of recognition to physiotherapists who complete advanced training. Canada and the United States offer registration to physical and occupational therapy members of the American Hippotherapy Association who complete a minimal amount of advanced training. AHA registration, however, is not a statement of proficiency but simply an indication that a therapist has completed training in hippotherapy. Brazil offers one course each year to licensed therapists and physicians and reported the participation of Argentinean equotherapists in a recent Association Nacional de Equoterapia (ANDE) course (Cirillo, 1994). Israel has an elaborate educational program for riding instructors and therapists that is university based, leads to a diploma, and usually takes 2 years to complete. Australia offered its first course to Australian and New Zealand physiotherapists in November 1994, but at this time has no method of registering, certifying, or licensing therapists. England requires physiotherapists to take the Association of Chartered Physiotherapists of Riding for the Disabled (ACPRD) course, Horse in Rehabilitation, Parts I and II, which contains a hippotherapy component. England reports holding one hippotherapy training workshop for 12 physiotherapists currently practicing hippotherapy. Ireland requests that physiotherapists working in hippotherapy programs complete Part II of the ACPRD course.

Hippotherapists from several countries have taught workshops internationally, which have helped develop a broader understanding of therapeutic techniques. During the last 10 years, Austrian, German, and Swiss hippotherapists have taught courses in Europe and North America, and since 1990, hippotherapists from Canada and the United States have taught courses in Australia, Israel, and New Zealand.

In addition to special courses and training in horse handling required of hippotherapy practitioners, many countries list prerequisites for individuals prior to entering advanced training. For example, Austria requires its applicants to be trained in neurodevelopmental treatment or to have a minimum of 2 years of physiotherapy experience after receiving a diploma, plus 2 years of experience in a neurological treatment setting. Proficiency in dressage is also required.

Nearly all the European nations recognize levels of horsemanship with standard qualifications for each level. In countries with defined levels of riding competency, it is fairly easy to require physiotherapists to reach a certain level of training on and with the horse as part of their hippotherapy license or certificate. This is not true in many of the other nations, however. For example, in the United States, riding instruction is still a free-enterprise occupation with no examination of skill needed to qualify and little regulation imposed. This makes it difficult to require that therapists have a well-defined, standard level of competency with the horse prior to practicing hippotherapy. It is generally accepted, however, that physiotherapists who wish to work with clients in hippotherapy must be able to demonstrate certain riding and horse-handling skills.

Program Elements

In countries practicing hippotherapy, the clientele treated is varied. Clients with the diagnoses of cerebral palsy and multiple sclerosis are commonly served, especially in Austria, Germany, and Switzerland, where hippotherapy for persons with these diagnoses is readily accepted by third-party payers or insurance systems (Heipertz et al., 1981; Künzle, Egli, & Yasikoff, 1994). Data from a 1994 study (Heipertz-Hengst, 1994) characterize the diagnosis for hippotherapy clients served in German-speaking countries as cerebral palsy (26.6%), orthopedic problems (20.3%), multiple sclerosis (18.8%), posttraumatic spasticity (18.8%), and hyperkinetic syndrome (15.5%).

In other countries such as Australia, Canada, Israel, and the United States, any person with a neurologically based movement dysfunction could potentially qualify for hippotherapy. This includes persons with cerebral palsy and multiple sclerosis but also encompasses clients with traumatic brain injury, cerebral vascular accident, scoliosis, genetic syndromes, and developmental delay. Rather than list specific disabling neurological illnesses or conditions, however, the trend in hippotherapy treatment is to refer to it as a treatment for children and adults with mild to severe movement dysfunctions or disorders (American Hippotherapy Association, 1995).

Other data requested in the international survey were estimates of the number of clients receiving hippotherapy in a year. Most respondents indicated that accurate numbers were not available; estimates, however, ranged from 3,000 clients per year (Germany), to 500 (Brazil and the United States), to less than 40 in Australia, Belgium, Hong Kong, and Ireland.

Before treatment for any condition can be initiated, a prescription for hippotherapy from the client's physician is needed. Once the prescription is received and the entrance forms required by the hippotherapy program are completed, the therapist can schedule an evaluation of the client off the horse. If the evaluation indicates that the client is a candidate for hippotherapy, the equine-based treatment program is planned and initial goals are established.

Although it is essential that a specially trained physiotherapist—in some countries, this is extended to include occupational therapists—is the primary provider of hippotherapy, additional personnel are needed to complete the hippotherapy team. A skilled horse handler is required for a successful treatment session. The therapist sets the client goals and decides how the client and horse will interact to achieve those goals. The therapist also directs the horse handler who, through the use of long lines or a lead rope, influences the horse's movement to accomplish the desired transfer of motion from the horse's back to the client. In addition to the horse, the client, the therapist, and the horse handler, volunteer assistants may be needed to walk next to mounted clients to provide stability and ensure safety. It may also be desirable to include a psychologist, special educator, or speech therapist on the treatment team, depending on the client's needs. For example, ANDE of Brazil always includes a psychologist on its technical interdisciplinary team for hippotherapy, and in Belgium and the United States, speech therapists conduct treatment sessions.

Before the therapy team can begin, a safe environment is needed. Generally, this is an indoor riding ring with special footing. The area must be free of distractions. Variations used by different practitioners include fenced outdoor riding rings and the long straight walkway preferred in Hippotherapy-K. The ideal horse for hippotherapy is almost of mythical proportions. When a group of therapists discuss the characteristics of a suitable therapy horse, several necessary qualities always arise—and then a long list of "wouldn't it be nice if" qualities. Therapeutic riding horses in general must possess a gentle, tolerant temperament and be in good health. In addition, it is essential that a hippotherapy horse

- Be symmetrical and well-balanced
- Move with even strides and be capable of tracking up at the walk
- Be supple and well muscled
- Be trained to work on the bit, with a rounded frame, good impulsion, and smooth transitions

Breed, conformation, size, and its relationship to movement, plus training and horse care, are the subjects of articles, books, and workshops. Twelve countries reported providing special training to horses used in hippotherapy, whereas seven countries indicted they provide the same level of training for the horses used in all types of therapeutic riding. Additional study and experience with horses are essential for anyone wishing to practice hippotherapy (Engel, 1992; Harris, 1993; Heipertz et al., 1981; Schusdziarra & Schusdziarra, 1978; Spink, 1993a, 1993b; Strauss, 1991).

Once a client is accepted and evaluated, the horse and tack are chosen, the therapy team is assembled, and the treatment goals are set, the treatment session can begin. Each hippotherapy program has a designated mounting area with a mounting ramp or block. A gradually sloping ramp leading to a level platform is ideal and is considered essential if patients in wheelchairs are being served. The client is brought to the mounting ramp or block and assisted onto the waiting horse. Generally, the client sits upright facing forward. The therapist directs the horse handler and assistants, and the session begins when the horse handler prompts the horse to walk away from the mounting ramp to the designated treatment area. Once at the treatment area, how the horse moves at the walk depends on the therapy goals for the individual being treated. Options include a slow or brisk walk, with the horse collected or on a long rein; circles to the left or right and of varying diameter; gentle or quick stops and starts; figures-of-eight; and, if the horse is trained in dressage and capable of smooth transitions, serpentines, shoulder in, and leg-yielding maneuvers. As mentioned previously, the size, girth, and breed of the horse chosen for the treatment session can play a significant role in the amplitude and force of movement transferred to the client (Anthony, 1994; Jagielski, 1992).

While the horse and client are moving and being moved, the unique benefits of hippotherapy occur. The client's center of gravity shifts in response to the movement of the walking horse's back and produces accommodating muscular responses in the client. According to Tauffkirchen, in her 1992 presentation at the Sixth International Congress on Animals and Us, "The three dimensional motion coming from the back of the walking horse affects the sitting patient and provokes a reactive sitting pattern" (p. 124). Weber et al. (1994) documented changes in client's balance with studies using electromyography to chart muscle response.

Sessions vary from brief introductory periods of 10 to 15 minutes to sessions of 30 or even 60 minutes, depending on the tolerance of the client. The average duration of a typical hippotherapy session in our experience is 30 to 40 minutes. The number of clients treated varies from a one-on-one treatment session to a maximum of eight in the ring simultaneously in Norway.

When the client dismounts, it is important that the gains in posture, mobility, and balance be maintained and that the client transfer these gains into significant functional activities. The therapist may wish to continue the treatment for a short period after dismounting to reinforce the gains made while on the horse (Glasow, 1985).

Reimbursement for hippotherapy differs in each country surveyed. Twelve countries report some type of eligibility for insurance payment for certain clients. Eight countries have no organized way of paying for hippotherapy and vary from providing services free of charge to charging clients the equivalent of a regular riding session for able-bodied riders. In two instances, the therapists are paid directly by the country and, therefore, do not bill clients individually. Most respondents concur that recognition of hippotherapy as a medical service reimbursable by established insurance systems is desirable and that conformity of service for selected categories of patients is essential to achieve this goal.

Research

Country respondents were also asked whether any research has been conducted in their organization to assess the benefits of hippotherapy. Of the respondents, 10 answered yes and 11 no. International conferences on therapeutic riding have been conducted since 1974, with hippotherapy as a prominent presentation topic. Of the 10 nations who responded that research has been conducted, all have sent representatives to international conferences, and the papers they presented are published in conference proceedings (*Proceedings,* 1976, 1979, 1982, 1985, 1988, 1991, 1994). To date, Germany has published the greatest number of scientifically recognized research studies regarding the efficacy of hippotherapy. The *Deutsches Kuratorium für Therapeutisches Reiten quarterly journal, Therapeutisches Reiten,* lists 37 published articles from 1992 to 1994 with 10 of these articles referring to hippotherapy in their titles. Other countries with known published research material pertaining to hippotherapy include Switzerland, Austria, Italy, and Belgium (Tauffkirchen, 1993; Veicsteinas, Melorio, & Sarchi, 1994). Finland, France, and the United States responded yes to having completed research, but Finland and France did not include published references, and the United States studies are pending publication. Brazil, England, and Israel reported one or more studies in progress.

In a two-phase study reported at the 8th International Therapeutic Riding Congress, Heipertz-Hengst (1994) sought to assess the effects of hippotherapy in the dynamic and complex somatic, functional, and psychosocial areas. She developed a standard starting assessment form in a pilot study in 1989 and upgraded the assessment form in a second pilot study in 1993. Her goal is a standard client assessment performed before and after hippotherapeutic treatment. This standardized assessment approach permits a computerized statistical analysis of the benefits of hippotherapy treatment.

Engelmann (1994) reported that in 153 traumatically caused para- and tetraplegic patients with spasticity, hippotherapy resulted in a significant reduction of spasticity in 105 patients for periods from 2 to 36 hours. Many published research studies have been conducted on the effects of therapeutic riding and hippotherapy with patients with multiple sclerosis, cerebral palsy, and autism (Bertotti, 1988; Biery & Kauffman, 1989; Conway, Mackay-Lyons, & Roberts, 1988; Copeland Fitzpatrick, 1994; Künzle et al., 1994; Weber, 1994). In a 12-week study, Haehl (1996) explored the kinematic relationship between the horse and two riders with cerebral palsy. She used the dynamical systems approach to examine the influence of hippotherapy on the postural control of the rider, the Peak Performance System of videographics to digitize the riders' sessions, and the Pediatric Evaluation of Disability Inventory to asses the participants' functional performance. Haehl's study demonstrates how to identify and measure the control parameters of postural orientation and postural stability and relate these to functional performance.

As hippotherapy continues to define its practice realm and technique, it is important that its theoretical base be examined. A theoretical framework is imperative in therapeutic riding as it evolves from practicing technicians applying techniques to professionals who base programs on a foundation of testable hypotheses and research data. DePauw (1992) calls for studies to examine the "human-horse-environment interaction" and suggests that this include "the three-dimensional movement of the horse, sensory stimulation and its integrative effects, and the horse-human bond" (p. 44).

The world is demanding functional results from the dollars spent on therapy. According to Stuberg and Harbourne (1994), "the emphasis of treatment has shifted from treating primarily the sequelae of the underlying pathology such as limitation of range of motion, weakness, or incoordination of movement to the utilization of a functional outcome framework" (p. 119). The latest concepts of motor development, motor control, and motor learning with the new knowledge of central nervous system function demand that contemporary theory be applied to treatment. Work on applying dynamic systems theory and its relation to motor control and learning to hippotherapy has been reported (Copeland, 1991; Copeland Fitzpatrick, 1994; Haehl, 1994, 1996; McGibbon, 1994). Haehl (1996) suggests that 10 subsystems are involved in the development of postural control, including coordinated movement patterns (synergies), visual, vestibular, and somatosensory systems for detecting loss of balance (feedback), anticipatory processes that pretune sensory and motor processes for posture in anticipation of potentially destabilizing tasks (feedforward), and adaptive systems for modifying sensory and motor systems to changes in task or environment. She states that "hippotherapy uses the movement of the horse to assist the rider in self-organizing these subsystems to form new coordinated movement patterns of postural control" (p. 31).

Heipertz-Hengst (1994) and Klüwer (1994) reported on instruments developed to help therapists gather data to determine outcome effectiveness with the hope that these data collection instruments will experience widespread use with reporting that can be statistically analyzed. Videographic techniques and gross motor statistical measures are becoming available, which can more readily be used with special populations. These instruments can assist in determining baseline and posttreatment performance (Haley, 1994). The North American Riding for the Handicapped Association Research Committee plans a meeting between the committee and the Board of Federation of Riding for the Disabled International at the Denver 1997 International Congress of Therapeutic Riding to discuss the development of an international database.[1]

The international practice of hippotherapy has taken giant strides toward defining itself, delineating its parameters, developing educational programs, and documenting results. In a world connected by communications networks, obtaining information has become fast and affordable. Through conferences, publications, and the Internet, all practicing hippotherapists can have access to case studies, research information, and educational activities offered by colleagues.

Hippotherapy needs the support of additional research. Efficacy for this unique medical treatment methodology is, and will ultimately be, based on scientifically conducted studies of significantly large enough samples. Hippotherapy's ability to effect long-term functional changes in clients must be documented through investigations that compare the results of hippotherapy to alternative therapies. The publication of such studies in recognized journals, books, and proceedings continues to support hippotherapy as a credible, internationally recognized, therapeutic treatment option.

Note

1. Contact names and addresses for the member countries may be obtained from the following:

> President, American Hippotherapy Association, North American Riding for the Handicapped Association, P.O. Box 33150, Denver, CO 80233
> President, Federation of Riding for the Disabled International, Am Zaarshäuschen 22, 51427 Bergisch Gladbach, Germany

References

American Hippotherapy Association. (1995). *Overview curriculum.* Denver, CO: North American Riding for the Handicapped Association.

Anthony, C. (1994). A walk that works. *Equus, 211,* 34-40.

Armstrong-Esther C., Sandilands, M., Myco, F. M., & Miller, D. (1988). Validation of horse riding as a therapy for physically and mentally handicapped adults. In *Proceedings of the 6th International Therapeutic Riding Congress* (pp. 1-43). (Information available through H. Brcko, 19 Alcaine Court, Thornhill, Ontario, Canada L3T 2G8)

Baillie, J. (1985). Where do we go from here? In *Proceedings of the 5th International Therapeutic Riding Congress* (pp. 191-194). (Information available through ANIRE, Via Triencea delle Frascag 2, 20136 Milan, Italy)

Baker, E. (1994). Precautions and contraindications to therapeutic riding: A framework for decision-making. In *Proceedings of the 8th International Therapeutic Riding Congress* (pp. 70-72). Levin, New Zealand: National Training Resource Center.

Bertotti, D. (1988). Effect of therapeutic horseback riding on children with cerebral palsy. *Physical Therapy, 68*(10), 1505-1512.

Biery, M., & Kauffman, N. (1989). The effects of therapeutic horseback riding on balance. *Adapted Physical Activity Quarterly, 6*(3), 221-229.

Britton, V. (1991). *Riding for the disabled.* London: B. T. Batsford.

Brown, O., & Tebay, J. (1994). *Directory of education and training: Federation of Riding for the Disabled International* (3rd ed.). Riderwood, MD: Therapeutic Riding Services.

Cawley, R., Cawley, C., & Retter, K. (1993). Therapeutic horseback riding and self-concept in adolescents with special educational needs. *Anthrozoös, 7*(2), 129-134.

Cirillo, L. (1994). Brazilian project on equotherapy. In *Proceedings of the 8th International Therapeutic Riding Congress* (pp. 181-183). Levin, New Zealand: National Training Resource Center.

Cohen, B. (1992, August 13). Therapy is key word in equine treatment. *Advance: The Physical Therapy Weekly,* 8, 48.

Conway, C., Mackay-Lyons, M., & Roberts, W. (1988). Effects of therapeutic riding on patients with multiple sclerosis: A preliminary trial. *Physiotherapy Canada, 40*(2), 12-14.

Copeland, J. (1991). A challenge to therapeutic riding. *Anthrozoös, 4,* 210-211.

Copeland, J. (1992) Three therapeutic aspects of riding for the disabled. In B. Engel (Ed.), *Therapeutic riding programs: Instruction and rehabilitation* (pp. 19-20). Durango, CO: B. Engel Therapy Services.

Copeland Fitzpatrick, J. (1994). The role of riding therapy in the treatment of spastic cerebral palsy following selective posterior rhizotomy. In *Proceedings of the 8th International Therapeutic Riding Congress* (pp. 5-6). Levin, New Zealand: National Training Resource Center.

Davies, J. A. (1988). *The reins of life.* London: J. A. Allen.

DePauw, K. (1992). Review of research in therapeutic riding. In B. Engel (Ed.), *Therapeutic riding programs: Instruction and rehabilitation* (pp. 43-45). Durango, CO: B. Engel Therapy Services.

Engel, B. T. (Ed.). (1992). *Therapeutic riding programs: Instruction and rehabilitation.* Durango, CO: B. Engel Therapy Services.

Engel, B. T. (Ed.). (1994). *Bibliography of the Federation of Riding for the Disabled International.* Durango, CO: B. Engel Therapy Services.

Engelmann, A. (1994). Hippotherapy results at paraplegic patients. In *Proceedings of the 8th International Therapeutic Riding Congress* (pp. 242-244). Levin, New Zealand: National Training Resource Center.

Glasow, B. (1985). Principles of NDT and normal development applied to hippotherapy progressions. In *Proceedings of the 5th International Congress Therapeutic Riding*. (Information available from ANIRE, Via Triencea delle Frascag 2, 20136, Milan, Italy)

Haehl, V. (1994). A dynamic systems approach to the use of hippotherapy. *American Hippotherapy Association News, 3,* 1-4.

Haehl, V. (1996). *Exploring the influence of hippotherapy on the kinematic relationship between the rider and the horse.* Unpublished master's thesis, University of North Carolina, Chapel Hill.

Haley, S. M. (1994). Our measures reflect our practices and beliefs: A perspective on clinical measurement in pediatric clinical physical therapy. *Pediatric Physical Therapy, 6,* 142-143.

Harris, S. (1993). *Horse gaits, balance and movement.* New York: Macmillan.

Heipertz, W., Heipertz, C., Kröger, A., & Kuprian, W. (1981). *Therapeutic riding* (M. Takeuchi, Trans.). Stuttgart, Germany: Kosmos Verlag.

Heipertz-Hengst, C. (1994). Evaluation of outcome in hippotherapy. In *Proceedings of the 8th International Therapeutic Riding Congress* (pp. 217-221). Levin, New Zealand: National Training Resource Center.

Jagielski, C. (1992). Techniques of long-reining during hippotherapy and therapeutic riding sessions. In B. Engel (Ed.), *Therapeutic riding programs: Instruction and rehabilitation* (pp. 119-137). Durango, CO: B. Engel Therapy Services.

Joswick, F., Kittredge, M., McCowan, L., McParland, C., & Woods, S. (1986). *Aspects and answers.* Augusta, MI: Cheff Center for the Handicapped.

Klüwer, B. (1994). Psychomotoric movement: Observation in hippotherapy. In *Proceedings of the 8th International Therapeutic Riding Congress* (pp. 79-87). Levin, New Zealand: National Training Resource Center.

Klüwer, C. (1988). The specific contribution of the horse in different branches of therapeutic riding for the disabled. In *Proceedings of the 6th International Therapeutic Riding Congress* (pp. 268-294). (Information available through H. Brcko, 19 Alcaine Court, Thornhill, Ontario, Canada L3T 2G8)

Klüwer, C. (1992). The Federation of Riding for the Disabled International. In B. Engel (Ed.), *Therapeutic riding programs: Instruction and rehabilitation* (pp. 27-29). Durango, CO: B. Engel Therapy Services.

Klüwer, C. (1994). Some considerations regarding the development of the Federation Riding for the Disabled International. In *Proceedings of the 8th International Therapeutic Riding Congress* (pp. 165-167). Levin, New Zealand: National Training Resource Center.

Kröger, A. (1992). Using vaulting lessons as "remedial education." In B. Engel (Ed.), *Therapeutic riding programs: Instruction and rehabilitation* (pp. 609-617). Durango, CO: B. Engel Therapy Services.

Künzle, U. (1995, September). *Hippotherapy-K: The use of the horse in physiotherapy* [Abstract]. Paper presented at the 7th International Conference on Human-Animal Interactions: Animals, Health, and Quality of Life, Geneva, Switzerland.

Künzle, U., Egli, R. S., & Yasikoff, N. (1994). Hippotherapy-K: The healing rhythmical movements of the horse for patients with multiple sclerosis. In *Proceedings of the 8th International Therapeutic Riding Congress* (pp. 63-69). Levin, New Zealand: National Training Resource Center.

La thérapie avec le cheval: Historique et methodologie [Brochure; Therapy with the horse: History and methodology]. (1995). Vincennes, France: Association Pour La Spécialisation, L'Enseignement et la Recherche dans les Thérapeutiques D'Approche Corporelle. (Available from the Association, 21 rue Massue, Vincennes, France 94300)

Leimer, G. (1993). Indikationen von heilpädagogischem voltigieren und reiten bei anorexia nervosa [Indications for remedial vaulting and riding for anorexia nervosa]. *Therapeutisches Reiten, 22,* 10-13.

McGibbon, N. (1994). Motor learning: The common denominator. In *Proceedings of the 8th International Therapeutic Riding Congress* (pp. 63-69). Levin, New Zealand: National Training Resource Center.

North American Riding for the Handicapped Association. (1993). *NARHA guide.* Denver, CO: Author.

Proceedings of the 2nd International Therapeutic Riding Congress. (1976). (Information available through U. Künzle, Swiss Group for Hippotherapy-K®, Neurological University Clinic, 4031 Basel, Switzerland)

Proceedings of the 3rd International Therapeutic Riding Congress. (1979). (Information available through National Agriculture Centre, Kenilworth, Warwickshire, CV8 2LY, UK)

Proceedings of the 4th International Therapeutic Riding Congress. (1982). (Information available through Deutsches Kuratorium für Therapeutisches Reiten, e.V., Freiherr von langen Str. 13, 48231 Warendorf, Germany)

Proceedings of the 5th International Therapeutic Riding Congress. (1985). (Information available through ANIRE, Via Triencea delle Frascag 2, 20136 Milan, Italy)

Proceedings of the 6th International Therapeutic Riding Congress. (1988). (Information available through H. Brcko, 19 Alcaine Court, Thornhill, Ontario, Canada L3T 2G8)

Proceedings of the 7th International Therapeutic Riding Congress. (1991). (Information available through Dansk Handicap Idraets-Forbund, Idraettens hus, Brøndby stadion 20, 2605 Brøndby, Denmark)

Proceedings of the 8th International Therapeutic Riding Congress. (1994). Levin, New Zealand: National Training Resource Center.

Riede, D. (1986). *Therapeutisches reiten in der kranken-gymnastik* [Therapeutic riding (within the context of) physical therapy]. Munich, Germany: Pflaum-Verlag.

Riede, D. (1988). *Physiotherapy on the horse.* (A. Dusenburg, Trans.). Renton, WA: Delta Society. (Original work published 1986)

Riding for the Disabled Association. (1984). *RDI handbook* (3rd ed.). Kenilworth, Warwickshire, UK: Author.

Rosenzweig, M. (1987). Horseback riding: The therapeutic sport. In M. E. Berridge & G. R. Ward (Eds.), *International perspectives on adapted physical activity* (pp. 213-219). Champaign, IL: Human Kinetics.

Scheidhacker, M. (1994a). *Die arbeit mit dem pferd in psychiatrie und psychotherapie* [Working with the horse in psychiatry and psychotherapy]. Warendorf, Germany: Schnell, Buch & Druck.

Scheidhacker, M. (1994b). No pretension to being cured—but softening of symptoms and improvement of the quality of life. In *Proceedings of the 8th International Therapeutic Riding Congress* (pp. 97-99). Levin, New Zealand: National Training Resource Center.

Schusdziarra, H., & Schusdziarra, V. (1978). *An anatomy of riding.* Briarcliff, NY: Breakthrough.

Spink, J. (1993a). *Developmental riding therapy: A team approach to assessment and treatment.* Tucson, AZ: Therapy Skill Builders.

Spink, J. (1993b). *The therapy horse: A model for standards competencies.* Charlottesville, VA: New Harmony Institute.

Strauss, I. (1991). *Hippotherapie* [Hippotherapy]. Stuttgart, Germany: Hippokrates Verlag.

Strauss, I. (1993). Documentation of hippotherapy. *Therapeutisches Reiten, 21,* 20.

Stuberg, W., & Harbourne, R. (1994). Theoretical practice in pediatric physical therapy: Past, present, and future considerations. *Pediatric Physical Therapy, 6,* 119-125.

Tauffkirchen, E. (1992, August). *Hippotherapy of cerebral palsy children.* Paper presented at the Sixth International Conference on Animals and Us, Montreal, Quebec, Canada.

Tauffkirchen, E. (1993, March). Der gute Sitz auf dem Pferd: Voraussetzung für eine wirksame Hippotherapie [A good seat on the horse: A prerequisite for viable hippotherapy]. *Therapeutisches Reiten, 20,* 9-11.

Tebay, J., Rowley, L., Copeland, J., & Glasow, B. (1988). Training physical and occupational therapists as hippotherapy specialists. In *Proceedings of the 6th International Therapeutic Riding Congress.* (Information available through H. Brcko, 19 Alcaine Court, Thornhill, Ontario, Canada L3T 2G8)

Veicsteinas, A., Melorio, G., & Sarchi, P. (1994). Energy requirement and cardiorespiratory readjustment during therapeutic horse riding in disabled. In *Proceedings of the 8th International Therapeutic Riding Congress* (pp. 231-241). Levin, New Zealand: National Training Resource Center.

Weber, A. (1994, May). Hippotherapie bei multiple-sklerose-patienten [Hippotherapy of multiple sclerosis patients]. *Therapeutisches Reiten, 21,* 16-19.

Weber, A., Pfotenhauer, M., David, E., Leyerer, U., Rimpau, W., Aldridge, D., Reissenweber, J., & Fachner, J. (1994). Registration and evaluation of effects of hippotherapy with patients suffering from multiple sclerosis by means of electromyography and acceleration measurement. In *Proceedings of the 8th International Therapeutic Riding Congress* (pp. 231-241). Levin, New Zealand: National Training Resource Center.

PART II

Beyond Health: Extending the Definition of Health to Quality of Life

Cindy C. Wilson
Dennis C. Turner

Quality of life (QL) is a multidimensional construct that specifically extends the World Health Organization's (1947) definition of health to consider individuals' perceptions of their health and well-being, work, and finances. Wilson proposes a QL framework for evaluating potential benefits of human-animal interactions (HAI). Under this rubric, methodological issues are considered and alternative approaches suggested. The strength of this practical approach to measurement is the ability of researchers and program evaluators to use measurement tools with validity and reliability that are available in the literature. A longtime weakness of HAI research has been its propensity to create instruments for each study, rather than use previously constructed tools that would allow aggregation and eventually norming of data to occur. Commenting on Chapter 4, Allen states that the model should be tested with theoretical constructs from our own disciplines. In addition, studies should be assessed with a set of common instruments as exemplary means to restructuring and maximizing the potential of a national QL-HAI research agenda. Barofsky and Rowan present selected theoretical issues underlying QL and then suggest models of QL assessment that have great promise for the field. To date, there has been no attempt to assess HAI under a cognitive model. This approach holds great promise for future endeavors and fits well with the framework as described by Wilson.

References

World Health Organization. (1947). The Constitution of the World Health Organization. *World Health Organization Chronicle, 1,* 29. (Tech. Rep. Series 706)

A Conceptual Framework for Human-Animal Interaction Research 4

The Challenge Revisited

Cindy C. Wilson

Abstract

The potential benefit of the human-animal interaction has been explored for over 20 years with limited success. Continued concern focuses upon the reliance of anecdotal and case reports, as well as limited, well-designed empirical studies. Professionals from many disciplines have examined the benefit(s) a companion animal can have for persons with special needs. Pets can lower blood pressures (Baun, Bergstrom, Langston, & Thoma, 1984; Friedmann, Katcher, Thomas, Lynch, & Messent, 1983; Grossberg, Alf, & Vormbrock, 1988), heart rates (DeShriver & Riddick, 1990; Wilson & Netting, 1987), and anxiety (Wilson, 1991); enhance social environments (Brickel & Brickel, 1980-1981, Mugford & M'Comisky, 1975); and decrease depression (Bolin, 1987).

AUTHOR'S NOTE: The opinions contained herein are mine and do not necessarily reflect those of the Uniformed Services University of the Health Sciences or the Department of Defense. Portions of this chapter were presented at the 10th Annual Conference of the Delta Society, Portland, Oregon, October 1991, and the 7th Annual Meeting of the International Society of Pharmacoepidemiology, Basel, Switzerland, August 1991. This chapter is reprinted with permission from "A Conceptual Framework for Human-Animal Interaction Research: The Challenge Revisited," in *Anthrozoös*, Vol. 7, pp. 4-24, 1994.

Although much has been made over the potential benefits of a pet, little attention has been given to the key recommendations of the Delta Society Conferences in 1984 and 1986 and the NIH Technology Assessment Conference (1988), where participants proposed that theoretical bases of the various disciplines be adopted and tested in the area of human-animal interaction (HAI) research and studies be designed to include normal and non-normal populations of people, different cultures, nontraditional relationships, and those not interested in animals. Earlier recommendations have also been made to employ the use of a developmental (i.e., longitudinal) perspective (Wilson & Netting, 1987), allowing determination of benefit(s) of pet ownership over time. Optimally, pet owners and nonowners should be initially assessed at an early age and followed prospectively throughout their life span. An alternative, retrospective approach would be to identify coin parable cohorts, elicit historical data, measure present status, and follow each cohort for a specified time period. Both approaches are fraught with methodological limitations. A prospective approach is costly and often has a high attrition rate. The retrospective analysis is often biased by recall abilities.

The Predictive Model (Wilson & Netting, 1987) proposed a multivariable framework encompassing life course influencing variables, current circumstances, and outcome. Limited application of this model, the continued inability of researchers to quantify attitudes and attachment for a pet with clinical outcome measures, and the burgeoning segment of the population over age 65 led to a new proposal to assess potential benefit(s) of pet ownership.

This chapter presents a quality of life approach as a conceptual framework for evaluating potential benefit(s) to pet owners. Quality of life refers to clinically relevant aspects of subjective symptoms, feelings, and well-being. Measured by refined psychometric instruments that evaluate general well-being, subjective symptoms of mental/emotional status and functional and social status, quality of life represents an umbrella rubric under which the potential benefit(s) of the human-animal interactions can be analyzed. Methodological issues applicable to this approach include (1) who should assess quality of life, (2) what should be assessed, (3) how data should be used, (4) whether outcome measures should be generic or disease/dysfunction specific, (5) what are the time considerations for response scales, and (6) what psychometric properties should be considered in evaluation of questionnaires assessing quality of life. These issues will be addressed through the assessment of selected quantitative studies on human-animal interaction in light of the proposed quality of life approach.

Introduction

Much of the research on pet ownership and potential benefit to health remains anecdotal, nongeneralizable, and scientifically flawed (Marx, 1984). At the National Institutes of Health Technology Assessment Conference (NIH, 1988), several specific research areas were proposed to address issues of the potential health benefit of pets. These included the need to understand the benefit of pets in relationship to physical, mental, and social health of people. More specifically, conference participants concluded that pets have a special place in the environment and in the lives of people. Consideration of the potential benefit of a pet in the development of children and to the lives of older people cannot be overlooked,

Whatever benefits a companion animal may have for older people, whether real or perceived, require evaluation within the context of a conceptual framework. Previously, a life course developmental (i.e., longitudinal) perspective was proposed (Wilson & Netting, 1987) as a basis for evaluating research in the area. The usefulness of such an approach was in its ability to evaluate potential benefit(s) of pet ownership over a life span implied in previous research (Lago, Connell, & Knight, 1985) that indicates the importance of longitudinal rather than cross-sectional study. In addition, this model encompassed the areas of physical, mental, and social health perceived to be necessary in understanding potential benefits of ownership (NIH, 1988).

Life course development or continuity theory has been described as telling us that "as lives progress through time, a personal history is acquired. One's personal history becomes a variable in determining the pattern of subsequent life events" (Newman & Newman, 1984, p. 41). Thus, developmental approaches to evaluating human-animal interaction required some familiarity with studies completed with children, adolescents, and young adults. The literature in this area indicates that pets may reinforce self-esteem in preadolescent years (ages 9 to 12) because the pet can serve as a playmate/companion that communicates regard for its owner and fosters responsibility (Davis & Juhasz, 1985). Davis and Juhasz indicate that the pet's value as a developmental asset will fluctuate, depending on the individual needs, age, and sex of the owner. Therefore, the owner-pet bond is optimally a flexible affiliation from a developmental perspective, the healthy owner-pet relationship is evidenced by variability in attitudes and behavioral responses toward the pet over time. A rigid relationship indicates limitations in growth potential relative to developmental progress. (pp. 90-91)

Pets may represent different things to a person over time. A pet may serve as a confidant to the preadolescent but is less important during the adolescent years. As this "flexible affiliation" progresses, young adults often find their lifestyle limited by pet ownership demands. Those with young children often opt for ownership. Each person's life course becomes a pattern of adaptations that the person makes to the configuration of cultural expectations, resources, and barriers that exist during a particular period of time (Newman & Newman, 1984, p. 394). As people age, they make decisions, accept responsibilities, and reject some opportunities. Past experiences and decisions may influence choices (Newman & Newman, 1984). Theoretically, past experiences serve as indications of potential future relationships. If one's experience with pet ownership was positive, then the likelihood of incorporating a pet into one's environment may be higher than if one's previous experience with pets was negative.

With this perspective, Wilson and Netting (1987) proposed the Predictive Model as a life course development approach to predict potential benefit from pet ownership in the elderly. Based upon the Health Belief Model (Becker, 1974), the Predictive Model focused upon individual influences throughout the life course as well as individual perceptions (i.e., attitudes and attachments). The model comprised the life course predictors and current situational circumstances as operationalized through the following variables (Wilson & Netting, 1987):

Life Course and Influencing Variables

1. Ascribed characteristics such as sex, age, and ethnicity—variables one cannot control

2. Achieved characteristics such as socioeconomic status, educational level—variables that are "earned" during the life course and will influence "who one is" later in life

3. Former feelings about pets (i.e., a pet history), which include attitudes toward animals developed in earlier years, one's experience with pet ownership, and level of attachment toward previous pets

Current Circumstances

4. Housing variables—type of housing and occupancy

5. Health status—how one feels overall: physically, mentally, socially, economically, and environmentally

6. Current attitudes toward animals, pet ownership, level of attachment toward a pet, and time spent with a pet constitute this set of variables

Outcome

7. Individual well-being—how an individual responds to and hence potentially benefits from a pet depends on how the person perceives or values a pet

Conceptually, the Predictive Model (PM) provided a life course development framework for explaining previous inconclusive research data on benefits of pet ownership in community-based elderly. As a tool, the PM could predict potential benefit from pet ownership in the elderly based on individual influences throughout the life course as well as individual perceptions of attitudes and attachments toward a pet. Because the model was capable of evaluating both positive and negative "benefits" of a pet, it was useful in providing a rational explanation of various factors that have a part in the individual's life history, and thus why a pet intervention may or may not be appropriate.

However, there were limitations of this model. Instruments need to be refined or developed to measure the variables as described. Various scales have been used to assess individuals' attachment to their current or former pets (Friedmann, Katcher, Eaton, & Berger, 1984; Lago, Kafer, Delaney, & Connell, 1988; Ory & Goldberg, 1983; Poresky, Hendrix, Mosier, & Samuelson, 1987). The Pet Attitude Inventory (PAI) was specifically developed to measure pet history, attitudes, and attachments (Wilson, Netting, & New, 1985). In addition, the Animal Thematic Apperception Test (ATAT; Friedmann & Lockwood, 1991) has been developed to assess attitudes toward pets. However, limited use of these instruments has minimized the potential effectiveness of the Predictive Model. In addition, the complex nature of well-being as an outcome variable makes it difficult to dichotomize so that relationships between influencing variables and current circumstances can be assessed. Life events, intentional and unintentional, will not always be covered in this model. For example, sudden moves or changes in housing brought about by world events such as Desert Storm have caused families to move in ways that were not expected. Did these moves precipitate the loss of a beloved pet because of housing changes, or did the move provide the opportunity for the individual to obtain his or her first pet?

Limited application of the Predictive Model, the continued inability of researchers to easily quantify attitudes and attachment for a pet with clinical outcome measures, and the burgeoning segment of the population over the age of 65 led to this different conceptualization to assess potential benefit of pet ownership using a quality of life approach.

Quality of Life and the Human-Animal Interaction

Increasing attention is being focused upon the concept of quality of life and its relationship to clinical outcomes in a variety of settings. Health professionals involved in the care of cardiac, renal, long-term care, and other patients have expressed considerable interest in broadening the focus of therapeutic outcome measures beyond disease status (Hollandsworth, 1988) and survival (Levine et al., 1988). In 1984, a scientific study group of the World Health Organization suggested "loss of autonomy" as the end point in epidemiological studies of the relationships between specific diseases, disabilities, and dysfunctions. Although a key variable, the determination of "loss of autonomy" is subjective. The growing awareness of and interest in the subjective aspects of life quality following medical care or intervention has been described by Eiseman (1981) as part of the "length" versus "depth" issue. Eiseman notes, "There are those who, despite severe physical disabilities, live full, happy lives by any social, economic, philosophic, or emotional standards" (p. 11). Medical care may lengthen life, but medical, surgical, or pharmacologic therapies may reduce life quality by lengthy or multiple hospitalizations, intrusive or painful procedures, medications with adverse side effects, or interventions that are unwanted. There is concern not only with the length of life but also with positive elements that constitute the "qualities" that give life meaning and value. Subjective feelings about the quality of the life patients lead while undergoing therapy or treatment and while coping with chronic illness or disability are increasingly important when selecting and evaluating a treatment strategy. With elderly people experiencing at least one functional disability as they age and being at risk for other chronic conditions, the potential of a pet intervention bears examination as part of the quality of life.

Conceptual Basis for Quality of Life Measurements

 Historically, basic criteria for evaluation of new chemotherapeutic agents included classic indicators of therapeutic success (e.g., survival and objective response) as well as measures of performance, numbers of symptoms, improved mood, and a sense of well-being (Karnofsky & Burchenal, 1949). Today, many of these indicators would be classified as constituents of quality of life.

Quality of life assessments have been utilized to (1) describe the nature of functional and psychosocial problems associated with a condition, (2) establish norms for psychosocial morbidity among specific groups of people, (3) assess the efficacy of treatments and interventions, and (4) as a screening tool. However, an obvious limitation of the use and interpretation of QL data is the difficulty in reaching conceptual agreement of a definition of "quality of life" (Aaronson, 1989).

Subjective elements of quality of life have been measured repeatedly over the past 30 years. Extensive efforts by social scientists have been undertaken to define the constituent elements and the affective responses that denote QL (Andrews & Withey, 1976; Bradburn, 1969; Campbell, Converse, & Rodgers, 1976; Cantril, 1965; Flanagan, 1978). Based on the literature and potential usefulness of a pet intervention in HAI protocols, ten domains are suggested to define QL in study patients: (1) physical status and symptoms, (2) functional status, (3) role activities, (4) social activities, (5) emotional status, (6) cognition, (7) sleep and rest, (8) energy and vitality, (9) health perceptions, and (10) general life satisfaction/well-being. There is overlap between and among previous domains of QL and the life course influencing variables and current circumstances from the Predictive Model. However, the strength of the QL approach is that tools exist that are psychometrically sound in measuring respondent answers.

How to Measure QL

 How QL will be measured is related, in part, to its content conceptualization and in part to its organization along a continuum reflecting its application. Feinstein (1987) presents QL as an "umbrella" measure under which are placed many different indices dealing with various elements. The user is responsible for determining the specific focus of analyses. This allows the investigator to select appropriate measures for function, condition, or setting in which the assessment will be made. Quality of life may be measured by either a generic or global measure designed for use in a broad range of conditions or a specific intervention such as the use of a pet.

The strength of the global/generic class of measures is that they allow comparison of results across studies and with the calculation of quality adjusted life years (QUALYs). They may not, however, address topics of particular relevance for a specific disease, dysfunction, disability, or intervention. Conversely, more disease-specific measures lose generalizability to other conditions. Although there is great interest in the use of QUALYs by third-party payers, the numeric values generated may not be meaningful to clinicians or practitioners.

A different approach would be to use a single-item assessment that asks the respondents to evaluate their QL by answering the question, "How would you rate your QL today?" This single-item approach may be useful as a summary score in calculating QUALYs or rankings in a specific trial, but it too is limited in its interpretability.

Process Issues in the Quality of the Measurement: Validity, Reliability, and Responsiveness

Careful conceptualization of QL for use in human-animal interaction trial narrows the range of questions and instruments that could be used, but a relatively broad choice remains for how the questions are selected and validated. Validity is usually defined as the extent to which a test measures what it is intended to measure.

Most validation studies refer to content or face validity. Each measurement represents a sampling of questions from a larger number that could have been chosen. Content validity refers to the adequacy of the questions to reflect the aims of the instrument as specified by the conceptual definition of its scope. A common procedure to establish content validity is to ask experts to review the clarity and completeness of the questions as they are developed and tested.

After content validation, more formal statistical analysis is used to determine the level of validity of the measure. The simplest approach is to measure the concept in question against a "gold standard." This typically occurs when the new instrument is a simpler, shorter, or more convenient measure. The new and old measures are applied to an appropriate sample of people, and the results are compared using an appropriate correlation technique. This procedure is known as correlational, concurrent, or criterion validity. Unfortunately, without consensus on the conceptualization of QL as it relates to human-animal interaction, it is often difficult to identify criterion measures for comparative purposes.

An empirical means of establishing construct validity using a statistical technique is known as factor analysis. This approach examines the relationship of various items in an index of common elements. The approach is appropriately used when a measurement contains separate components, each reflecting a different aspect of QL. Patterns of intercorrelations among replies to questions form the questions into groups or "factors" that appear to measure common themes. Factor analysis, when used to assess the internal structure of an instrument rather than its correlation with other tests, is known as construct validity. The factor analysis approach was utilized in the development of an index to predict pet ownership in the military (Wilson, 1988).

Although an instrument may be valid, concern remains about the degree to which these scores can be replicated. In traditional measurement theory, the score obtained from any measurement is a combination of two components: an underlying score and some degree of error. Reliability is concerned with random error in measurements from respondents as well as the repeatability of results. The stability of a respondent rating is especially important when the measurement is compared over time; repeatability is estimated by applying the measurement two or more times and comparing the results, usually expressed as a correlation. These will be especially important values for future protocol developments in the field of human-animal interaction.

One of the issues related to quality of the instrument is how well it holds across various subject populations. It is generally recognized that the QL measure validated in a general population may not perform well when used in a hypertensive population. Likewise, there is some concern about the applicability in various age cohorts. Thus, expectations of potential benefit of a pet intervention will be different.

Other Measurement Issues: Who and When?

Historically, the physician has typically provided the QL assessment (Aaronson, 1989). This approach had two primary advantages: (1) It was less time intensive than interviewing subjects, and (2) in cases in which the subject is unable to provide QL ratings, physicians' ratings have, with caution, been used. However, data concerning performance standards indicate low levels of interphysician reliability and, more important, low levels of agreement between physicians and subjects (Hutchinson, Boyd, & Feinstein, 1979). Feedback from other providers and from family and friends may serve as complementary information but is no substitute for subject responses. In light of these data and the subjective elements of QL, it has been strongly argued that it is critical to directly interview subjects about the impact of the pet intervention on their daily lives.

Although there are technical issues related to the timing of a QL measure, assessments should, at a minimum, be made prior to and after the intervention. However, given the sensitive nature of individual responses, an interim measure is often needed. Wenger, Mattson, Furberg, and Elinson (1984) suggest serial assessments (i.e., at entry, annually, and at the end of a trial) and correlation with signs, symptoms, concurrent illness, and adverse effects. The ability to make multiple measurements is often a function of subject and project staff burden. An overly ambitious schedule of assessment may well result in missing data. Other time-related issues in the measurement of QL have to do with the time frame of the questions and the response scales utilized. It is often necessary to limit the time for obtaining information.

The provision of a specific reference point is also needed to orient the subject to time appropriately. For example, the use of a question "Do you tire more easily now than before you had a pet?" leaves the response open to a great deal of question. For the chronically ill or disabled person, the reference point is not clear, and subsequent data may not be relevant.

"Method" effects have received attention from the psychometricians. These effects represent a dependence of responses on the form and context of the question. Questions fall into two categories: (1) open-ended questions to which the respondent is free to make any response or (2) closed questions in which the respondent is supplied with a list of alternative responses or a fixed scale. Open-ended questions are less restrictive but more difficult to categorize and analyze. Closed questions tend to limit or force respondent answers.

Consideration should also be given to the means by which data are collected. Factors that should be considered include but are not limited to the mode of administration (i.e., direct observation, in-depth interview, etc.), scaling issues (i.e., content of the measurement and its level), aggregation of data, the complexity of scoring the data, and the distribution of scores.

Analyzing QL Data

Based on the times that data have been collected, data may be regarded as continuous. If forced choice responses have been used, data are categorical and often dichotomous. Analyses can be conducted under two main headings: description of the data collected and comparison of subjects in the different groups.

Questions that can be analyzed include: How many and which subjects have impaired QL? How long and how frequently has QL suffered? How severe is the impairment? How do these data relate to the pet intervention? If the data are continuous, simple descriptions are provided by estimates of location and changes over various time intervals. However, if the variable of interest is depression or anxiety, it is difficult to regard data presented as means and standard errors as informative measures. What does "average anxiety for the group" mean? If the data are discrete, they are reported as percentages that lead to pattern of change of various components of QL in an individual subject over time. Care must be taken to present the data in a logical and appropriate manner.

Selecting the Instrument

Data on changes in QL may provide additional information on the potential success of a pet intervention or program. Selection of the instrument(s) is a function of response variable identification. These variables will be determined by (1) the dysfunction or disability under study, (2) hypotheses to be tested and design of the experimental trial, (3) psychometric properties of the assessment tools, and (4) practical considerations of the project.

The investigator has three choices in the selection of the QL instrument: (1) use available, standardized instruments; (2) use clinical assessment; (3) custom design a new assessment instrument. Obviously, variants of these three alternatives are possible. For example, a series of items that measure an issue being evaluated in a specific study can be combined with the items on a standardized instrument, or standardized instruments can be rewritten for a specific setting (i.e., community-based vs. institutional setting). In either case, the psychometric properties of the instrument have been changed. The extent and scope to which the instrument matches the goals and objectives of the study are important. If an instrument selected for use in assessing the impact of a pet intervention in hypertensive subjects was originally utilized with coronary artery bypass patients, the functional consequences of the pet intervention may range from minimal to extreme. If the assessment instrument is designed to assess a wide range of functional outcomes but there is minimal consequence of the particular disease and intervention being studied, it is probably not useful to use such an instrument. It would lack specificity, and composite scores would not differentiate any quality of life effects of the pet. The chance acceptance of the null hypothesis when it is false (Type II error) would be increased.

To date, more than 83 different instruments have been utilized to measure QL (Hollandsworth, 1988). Of these 83 instruments, approximately 68 attempt to present elements of psychometric properties (i.e., reliability and validity). Thus, the selection of the instrument(s) is not always an easy one.

Implications of QL Trials and Human-Animal Interaction

Researchers have long hypothesized that pets can have a salutary effect on health by reducing anxiety (Wilson, 1991), loneliness, and depression (Friedmann, Katcher, Lynch, & Thomas, 1980; Katcher, 1981). Specific populations have shown positive benefit from pet interventions, among them the elderly (Garrity, Stallones, Marx, & Johnson, 1989; Stallones, Marx, Garrity, & Johnson, 1990), and children (Melson, 1990; Poresky et al., 1987). However, data from these studies are difficult to compare because of the differing methodologies, instruments, and conceptual frameworks. The quality of life approach is useful in its ability to measure a wide range of elements (i.e., the 10 domains of QL) with psychometrically sound tools and at the same time utilizing a theoretical framework that can be applied across populations, diseases, disabilities, or dysfunctions. Another strength is the ability to tie research hypotheses on the HAI benefit(s) to conceptual theory bases that are accepted within the various disciplines.

To date, none of the studies attempting to evaluate potential health benefit(s) of human-animal interaction has attempted to measure all domains of quality of life. Although understandable in part, this has left the studies open to criticism that any potential benefit found may be spurious and a factor related only to a specific cohort. The use of a conceptual framework such as QL provides insight into the very nature of the link between animals and humans. Major research questions that could be better addressed include (1) for whom is the animal interaction most beneficial and (2) what is the health "effect" of animal contact/intervention in the broadest sense? QL measures will continue to be used in a wide variety of decision making. Respondent perception of impact or satisfaction with level of well-being, dysfunction, or disability is a particularly important consideration in the final evaluation of the efficacious nature of any intervention. The use of a pet intervention in specific groups of people may well be guided by these data.

Comments

A Conceptual Framework for Human-Animal
Bond Research: The Challenge Revisited

Karen Allen, State University of New York at Buffalo,
197 Farber Hall, 3435 Main St., Buffalo, NY 14214

Somewhere in the corpus of the fairy tales surely there is a magical wizard who, with a wave of a wand, could quickly lead us to the most pragmatic and empirically sound way to unravel the mysteries of our relationships with animals. Until such a wizard appears, however, we must rely on mere mortal researchers to explain the human-animal bond, and over the past few decades, there has been no shortage of such research attempts. Although past conceptualizations of desirable approaches and methods concerning this field have had some merit, the Quality of Life Model presented by Wilson far surpasses earlier attempts and is an exceptionally thoughtful and practical approach to solving the problem confronting us.

My comments on the strengths and possible drawbacks of the Quality of Life Model as described by Wilson are based on a decade of careful observation of (1) trends of research in this field, (2) response of academic colleagues, as well as of the public, to the results of such research, and (3) the importance of sponsored research.

The most significant advantage of the Quality of Life Model is its conceptualization into ten domains that are possible to assess with existing measures. Also, because quality of life is of great importance to everyone, this model will be useful with all populations. However, though the model is exemplary, I fear that without further structure it will be disregarded in much the same manner as its predecessors (e.g., the Predictive Model).

Consequently, it appears that if we truly want to test the usefulness of this model, we should consider forming a research task force to come up with a consensus battery of psychometrically sound measures that could be recommended for each of the ten domains. Such a group of recommended measures could contribute to the ability to make comparisons between studies, improve the quality of the research, and improve the credibility of a fledgling field that has floundered long enough. Nothing would prevent prospective researchers from incorporating additional methods of assessment, but a common set of measures would provide a common ground for discussion. Also, a common set of measures would increase our abilities to do large-scale, multisite, collaborative research that could ultimately form a database of information about human-animal interaction.

My recommendation about common, standard measures is made partly to deal with the (often justified) criticism we hear from colleagues who see our investigations into our relationships with fluffy creatures as fluffy research. What makes our investigations different and subject to raised eyebrows and amused tolerance is the fact that most of us, if not all, are motivated by a love for our pets. We may be accomplished researchers with numerous advanced degrees and extensive publication lists, but we also have an emotional dimension in our research that makes us suspect in the eyes of our "serious" colleagues. To diminish this suspicion, we are going to have to develop an empirically sound, common research methodology that we all follow. The Quality of Life Model provides the perfect base upon which to build such a set of research principles. Just as we all learned and follow the methodologies of our respective fields, we can devise and learn to follow a common set of rules for studying the human-animal bond.

Far from perceiving such an approach as intrusive, my perception is that researchers would welcome a set of definitive guidelines. I believe that if we treat the study of quality of life as it relates to human-animal relationships as an applied area within each of our respective disciplines, we will do better research than if we try to create a new interdisciplinary field. If we combine suggestions from the 1988 NIH Technology Assessment Conference with elements of the Quality of Life Model, it appears that we will have a formula for success.

Specifically, we should explore various domains of quality of life within the context of theory testing in our own disciplines and use common measures for outcome assessment. Such an approach, combined with sound methodology, is a good strategy, and it is possibly the best way to gain credibility for the study of human-animal relationships. A formula that I recently found to be especially successful was to take two competing theories in my field and demonstrate how quality of life outcomes differed according to subjects' involvement with their pets. To add some spice to the study, my collaborator was a psychologist who believes that pets are totally useless! Such an approach allowed me to add to our understanding of human-pet interaction while simultaneously contributing to theory testing in social psychology and demonstrating that when another species is considered, perhaps some of our theories need to be rethought. It also enabled me to publish the findings in the leading journal in my field and finally be taken seriously in this area of my research. My colleagues may still call me "Dr. Woof," but they have to admit that I have done empirically sound, interesting work that just happens to be about pets! Finally, in addition to improving credibility and therefore attracting other researchers to this field, such a strategy dramatically increases chances of future funding for related research.

In conclusion, the Quality of Life approach as proposed by Wilson provides an exceptionally fine and realistic model for researchers who are intrigued by the possible meanings of animal-human relationships. It is likely that persuading researchers to follow this model with any degree of uniformity and structure will be a genuine challenge. If we meet this challenge, we will be able to begin to engage in research studies that will relate to each other in meaningful ways and collectively demonstrate sound evidence for the manner in which human-animal interaction is related to quality of life issues. If we choose not to meet this challenge, however, I fear we are doomed to a future of unrelated sound and fury that collectively says very little.

Conceptual Frameworks for Human-Animal Bond Research: A Commentary

Dan Lago, Ph.D., Associate Professor of Human Development and Health Education, College of Health and Human development, Penn State University, University Park, PA 16802

The Need for Conceptually Driven Research

The chapter by Cindy Wilson, and the emphasis it is receiving in the pages of this book, serve a valuable function for the scientific study of human-animal relationships, that is, timely reinforcement of the need to carefully design and conduct research studies to address particular questions raised by an explicitly stated conceptual model, or theory, of the human-animal relationship. From this foundation, all subsequent sampling, definition, and measurement procedures, and analysis decisions are made. More important, as "tests" of ideas on how the relationship works, such studies add more to our knowledge than casually defined studies.

As Wilson documents, each of the efforts to promote improved quality of human-animal relationship research has made specific reference to explicit theory development and to borrowing existing behavioral science theoretical models, such as family functioning, attachment theory, social relationship exchange theory, confidants and social support theory, etc. Despite these admonitions, research perspectives have not shown dramatic improvement. Thus the fact that any model is presented that specifies mediating factors and a range of outcome measures is to be applauded, rather than solely questioned in the details of how specific factors ought to be viewed.

Wilson's Life Course Model Makes Contributions

The major point of this model is that it emphasizes the dynamic nature of human-animal relationships in terms of the human's life stage. Equally useful may be to think in terms of variability during the stages of development of the human-animal relationship itself: the early rearing and bonding stage, active midlife, geriatric pet, etc. Because of life event changes, and attitudinal changes, the detailed behavioral activity patterns between an owner and a companion animal can show decided shifts over time, and the role of animal can change dramatically (for example, the pet in the new chronic disease household or bereaved household).

Second, Wilson necessarily emphasizes the need for longitudinal methods and suggests several different variants of designs that explicitly include the passage of time as a researchable dimension. This is very important in our opinion. Largely due to small-scale research resources, most studies of animal relationships are cross-sectional. We would underline Wilson's point about longitudinal data providing a different picture than cross-sectional. Results from various reports of our longitudinal study, the Companion Animal Project, with four points of measurement across seven years tend to support the idea of relationships being dynamic in one very important aspect: pet ownership. Cross-sectional results in year 1 did not show significant associations between pet affection attitudes and health benefits, but longitudinal findings over one year and over three years did show positive significant associations on both physical and especially mental health (Lago, Connell, & Knight, 1985; Lago, Delaney, Miller, & Grill, 1989; Lago, Knight, & Connell, 1983).

In the early years of our study, persons shifted between the "current owner" and "former owner" category, with approximately 10% in each category changing status. Later in the study (Lago et al., 1985; Lago et al., 1989), however, euthanizing old, ill pets and not getting new ones accounted for over 50% of the increasing number of current owners becoming "former owners." Another significant group had to surrender their pets in moving to a new residence, often a health care facility. At the end of our study, pet owners represented 38% of the sample, compared with 49% at the beginning. There was an increased rate of death among the former owner subgroup and a tendency for current owners to become former owners before death. Those current owners who had died by the time of our next follow-up study were significantly lower on the PRS scale [of] affectionate companionship than other current pet owners and had as a group experienced negative changes on their reported average level of "affectionate companionship." This reduction in average level of affectionate pet attitudes as death nears bears some similarity to traditional "disengagement" models in gerontology.

The emphasis on "quality of life" in Wilson's model is helpful. Quality of life outcomes, as a multidimensional array of variables, helps to clarify that there may be many different avenues through which pets may benefit people. In our opinion, a number of our measures can be viewed as outcomes within this quality of life rubric. Consistent with emphasis on affective bonds in the human-companion animal relationship, an emphasis on positive emotional tone and self-rated mental health seems reasonable, but emphasizing other dimensions of the human-animal relationship may shift emphases in outcome assessment to other areas. Thus for an individual who placed a great emphasis on her dog's "hearing-ear" help, social quality of life indicators would hopefully include monitoring the number of phone conversations held (since the phone was picked up), and nutritional status changes (due to hearing home meals staff, so that meals can be received), and home cleanliness (since cleaning aides were heard and admitted).

In multivariate research, this inclusive definition of quality of life does run the risk of confounding variables defined as baseline conditions, or mediating factors, with outcome measures. Thus an essential step in expanding and refining such a quality of life model is articulating how the earlier levels of quality of life independently continue to influence the outcome levels one obtains. The next two sections elaborate on this theme by discussing the role of two domains included in Wilson's model, but not in an elaborated way.

Health Status as a Critical Dimension

Overlap between mediating factors and outcome measures is most clearly displayed in the domain of health status. Physical health and functional status are contained within quality of life outcomes but also represent major predictors of outcome, depending upon their baseline level (Lago et al., 1989). Particularly among vulnerable, chronically ill populations, animal relationships may mean more than they do among the general population, who have increased options for the activities and companions they select in their attempts to achieve quality of life. Thus bonded relationships with pets may affect health outcomes interactively with current health status, benefiting primarily those in poorer health, but not in such poor health that they cannot manage the responsibilities of animal care. Our longitudinal and cross-sectional analyses among an elderly sample have consistently found health status measures as the strongest predictors of morale and well-being outcomes. This domain may be less important in some childhood or young adult samples, but any models used in investigations with any special, disabled, or aging populations should focus extensively on health status changes and impact on performance.

Other Human Social Relationships as a Context

Just as health status represents a complex domain of baseline, mediating, and outcome measures, so also does the complex array of human relationships (or the lack of them) that surround a particular human-animal relationship. This topic has been given lip service in a number of investigations but represents a major area of improved research and for much more carefully conceptualized theory. Whether pets serve as a "social substitute" or "supplement" or are essentially unrelated to human relationships probably varies dramatically for different individuals, depending on their changing expectations and social roles. An early analyses by our group (Connell & Lago, 1984) found different patterns of pets contributing to morale by marital status: for those who lived alone, pet affection was, positively associated with morale, for those who lived with a spouse, the highest levels of pet affection were negatively correlated with morale. Our most recent paper (Miller & Lago, 1990a) suggests that human social relationships are the primary nonhealth factor associated with emotional well- being and that the significant association of pet attitudes on emotional well-being is largely explained by the respondents' appraisal of their social support. As cited in our papers, a number of investigators have reported stronger associations of pet affection and high morale in people who are socially deprived in a way they deem important. Models of human-animal relationship need to explicitly include the human social context and specifically whether it is oriented toward supporting or downplaying the animal relationship.

How Broadly Should We Define
the Human-Animal Relationship?

A theme repeated in most of our publications is that current emphases on human-pet relationships as bonded, essentially affectionate emotion-laden interactions are too narrow for the complex array of different ways humans and pets relate. Andrew Rowan (1992) has recently commented on "the dark side of the force," those taboo, negative aspects of animal relationships that are usually not discussed even among researchers of human-animal relationships but that anecdotally do occur (neurotic and psychopathological relationships with pets, bestiality, cruelty, and abuse, etc.). Even more important than these aberrations, in our opinion, are the instrumental dimensions of animal assistance for certain owners and the strong value of pets or domestic animals for what they actually do, from the owner's perspective. Conceptual models of animal relationships are required that are broad enough to account for the emotional well-being and satisfaction of farmers/animal husbandry perspectives who report loving animals but use them in utilitarian ways, including eating, and still report that animals are a positive part of their quality of life.

In our opinion, affection for pets is too narrow a focus of measurement, and lack of powerfully significant results by many investigators in this area suggests that people who differ widely in how much they like pets can still find many different alternative paths to high-level quality of life; even people who score high on our measures of affectionate pet ownership still differ dramatically in how they may relate to animals.

For example, our recent study of a broad array of animal attitudes (including pet attitudes) with a random sample of adults (Kafer, Lago, Wamboldt, & Harrington, 1992) suggests that there are cohort and gender differences in self-report affection for pets. Further, some of the activities that are important in expressing affection among older women (feeding rituals and bathing the pet) do not appear to be important in the responses of a random adult population. Further, more utilitarian attitudes (that support food use, hunting, and experimentation, and in general require killing, "consumptive use") tend not to be held by those with the highest pet affection scores, but even though the correlations are substantial and significant, variable responses indicate that there are many in the sample who would display anomalous patterns of high pet affection and high utilitarian attitudes, or vice versa.

As an additional example, our observational data of affectionate pet owners and their pets in the home (Miller & Lago, 1990b) suggest that actual behavior of those high in self-report affection for pets shows extensive differences by species (dogs and cats). If there are physiological mechanisms by which animal relationships affect well-being (as strongly suggested by the handling and blood pressure studies), we should see more emphasis on differential impact of actual behavioral activities with pets and on details of the relationship and ultimately on well-being. Otherwise, we must adopt the somewhat surprising position that relationship content makes no difference, only how you think of it. This broader conception of the human-animal relationship explicitly requires more assessment effort and additional data beyond generalized self-reports of affection that have predominated in most early studies (see Kafer et al, 1992; Lago et al., 1988).

Conclusion

Increased research on the human-animal relationship is strongly merited, for basic reasons of increased understanding and for applied consequences related to both human and pet welfare. Preliminary findings have assured us that the topic is difficult to study and consequently that theoretical modeling and careful construction of research, especially with regard to sampling and measures, are required in order to produce useful findings. Given the arguments we have made, which generally call for nesting the animal companionship within a larger context, and the costs of conducting full-scale studies with the statistical power likely to produce significant findings, the strategies of linking animal companionship studies within other research still seems like a very sensible plan for most behavioral science researchers. For those with clinical settings and detailed information on small, but very interesting samples of persons, more intensive repeated measures designs should be employed to detect the effect of pets amid a series of other, ongoing effects.

Utilize What We Know

Martin B. Marx, Professor of Epidemiology, Emeritus,
University of Kentucky, College of Medicine, Lexington, KY 40536

I endorse the thoughtful way in which Dr. Wilson proposes her conceptual framework for future human-animal bond research. We all may wish for instruments that can accurately and precisely measure human emotions and assess a person's quality of life. Perhaps with more reliable and valid instruments, we could clarify for many subgroups of our population specific health effects that accompany strong attachment to a pet. This seems unlikely for two reasons.

First, instruments used in the social sciences are rarely valid or reliable enough to predict specific effects. They are usually intended to suggest very general hypotheses. Second, the relationships between human emotions and subsequent health effects are always complex, full of confounding variables, and in many cases, speculative. Therefore, they do not lend themselves to specific conclusions, especially those drawn from imprecise instruments.

Although Dr. Wilson's thoughtful description of the conceptual and methodologic issues involved in measuring QL is appreciated, I would prefer to build on what we already know from recent research. A great deal of very worthy research has been conducted since I wrote that harsh assessment of the early efforts on this subject (Marx, 1984). Indeed, Dr. Wilson has conducted some of it herself, as have Poresky, Samuelson, Hendrix, Mosier, Connell, Knight, Melson, and Lago, as well as Garrity, Marx, Stallones, Johnson, and many others. The quality of most of the work done by these researchers has been considerably more scientifically valid than the early anecdotes and case reports.

Much progress has been made, and a few associations between human health and pet attachment have been documented. These associations have been found rather consistently in very specifically defined groups. I can assure Wilson that the findings of the two national sample surveys conducted by the group with whom I was associated were conducted on correctly stratified national probability samples, with the specific intent of producing generalizable data.

In our first survey of persons 64 years and over (Garrity et al., 1989), the association between less depression and strong attachment to a pet was only demonstrable in elderly persons who suffered great distress, for example, the bereaved, and had few available confidants. That certainly makes sense and seems to me a contribution to a better understanding of the relationship.

In our second national survey of persons 21-64 years of age (Stallones et al., 1990), it was shown that pet ownership and attachment to pets did contribute to the overall model of illness behavior and emotional distress. This contribution was not consistent, but by its very inconsistency, it provided support for the notion that although selected population group[s] may benefit from pet ownership, the association between ownership, strong attachment, and human health is a complex and inconsistent one through all the age groups. It should be noted these associations were examined within the framework of the well-recognized theoretical model originally developed by Hans Selye, modernized by Thomas Holmes and Richard Rahe, and clearly delineated in our published research reports.

If further studies are indicated, and better instruments may be needed, I am concerned about who should contribute the study and control groups for validating the instruments, based on all the findings from recent research. I would want to know how the groups would be selected and exactly how "pet intervention" would be accomplished.

In summary, I respectfully take exception to Dr. Wilson's comments regarding our present state of knowledge of the relationship between human health and attachment to pets.

We know that salubrious effects have been documented in selected groups. We know from only the two surveys cited that the effects are not consistent throughout the various age groups and that the effects are complex and interwoven with confounding variables that relate to the degree of attachment one feels for the companion animal and the existence of other sources of support.

There are many areas of benightedness that cry out for more research. However, in the area of human-companion animal research, let us not "play the scientific game." First, let us utilize what we know. We should all read Bernard Rollin's (1988) comments in response to an earlier paper on human-animal bond theoretical underpinnings.

Reflections on a Quality of Life Model for Assessing Impact of Pets on Humans

Gail F. Melson, Department of Child and Family Studies, Purdue University, West Lafayette, IN 49707

The journal *Anthrozoös*, the annual conferences of the Delta Society, and the burgeoning number of articles appearing in journals of numerous disciplines all attest to a veritable explosion of research aimed at documenting the impact of contact with animals on human well-being. As a critical mass of evidence accumulates, increasing attention is now being paid to efforts at theoretical and conceptual integration (Melson, 1990). Cindy Wilson's "challenge," in her call to adapt a quality of life model to assessments of pet ownership and pet interventions, is an important contribution to the search for theoretical frameworks. Such frameworks are important for a number of reasons: (1) to provide guideposts for future research by generating testable predictions, (2) to develop a common vocabulary of measures so that findings from different studies may be compared, and (3) to link research on human-animal interaction with basic knowledge about human (and animal) functioning.

As Dr. Wilson states, the Quality of Life model (QL) is not intended to supplant alternate conceptualizations, such as the Predictive Model (Wilson & Netting, 1987). Rather, application of a QL framework is viewed as supplementary. Its principal benefit may lie in the availability of a variety of psychometrically sound measures to quantify "individual well-being" as an outcome. Within this framework, the impact of pet-related, or more broadly, animal-related experiences, may be more precisely measured and compared to the impact of other experiences. For example, for homebound elderly, the impact of an animal-visitation program might be compared with the impact of a home health care worker (human visitation only) on indices of general well-being, functional autonomy (i.e., ability to perform self-care tasks), or satisfaction with life.

Application of a QL model encourages researchers to view involvement with animals in the context of multiple social influences. Thus, the impact of pet ownership or interaction with animals in educational or therapeutic settings may be viewed not in isolation, but in interaction with other social influences. For example, involvement with animals may affect the quality of life of children or adults experiencing multiple stresses (from poverty, family dislocation, etc.) differently from those who are not highly stressed. An analogous pattern has been found for provision of human social support. Highly stressed children or adults appear to benefit more in terms of perceived quality of life from human social support than do those who are not experiencing much stress (Colletta & Lee, 1983; Unger & Powell, 1980). This raises the question of whether quality of life effects of pet ownership or other experiences with animals may vary for different individuals, depending on other aspects of their lives.

Thus, application of a QL model may be most fruitful for future research when pet ownership (or other animal-related experiences) is viewed as just one of many aspects of individuals' lives that must be measured. In practice, this approach makes it difficult to isolate the impact of interaction with or attachment to an animal from the context in which human-animal interaction occurs. For example, if an animal-visitation program results in increased QL scores for an institutionalized population, is this due to individuals' experiences with the animal "visitors" as many might assume? To what extent is QL improved by accompanying changes in staff mood or staff interaction? To disentangle these multiple and interacting effects on QL, research designs need to provide for appropriate control groups. When measuring the impact of pet ownership or bonding with a pet, it becomes even more difficult to isolate experiences with the pet from other contextual factors. Indeed, QL itself may be as much a determinant of pet bonding as an outcome. Individuals with better psychological functioning may be more able to develop and sustain caring relations with others, including animals. To determine effects of pet ownership on individuals, it is important to conduct longitudinal, prospective studies, in which changes in quality of life can be measured before and after developing a bond with a pet.

Documenting quality of life changes as a result of pet ownership or involvement with animals in other ways is an important challenge that researchers must meet in the decade of the 1990s. But even accomplishing this task will only raise further questions. What underlying processes account for quality of life changes (if found)? To demonstrate that owning a pet increases an elderly individual's sense of well-being does not explain how it does so. Is the effect produced by the sense of unconditional acceptance, by nurturing another, by feelings of attachment, by responsibility for another's well-being, and so forth? Examination of the processes by which animals affect human quality of life may well illuminate broader issues of human and animal well-being.

Author's Response: "A Conceptual Framework for Human-Animal Interaction Research: The Challenge Revisited"

Seeking a unified conceptual framework from which scientists from a broad array of interdisciplinary fields might collaborate in their research on human-animal interactions (HAI) is a means of generating renewed interest in the field. Moreover, it is an attempt to stimulate empirical research having a common thread in a more organized fashion.

Comments by reviewers suggest quality of life (QL) approach has merit because of (1) its ability to utilize existing reliable and valid measures that test an intervention (i.e., pet visitation/placement/ownership) within a structure that can be translated to a wide variety of disciplines (Melson; Allen; Lago); (2) its structure for theory testing within disciplines (Allen); and (3) its multidimensional nature, which allows the researcher to tease out the impact of a pet from other contextual differences (Melson; Lago). In addition, the QL approach fits well with the need for longitudinal studies as yet undone in the field of HAI (Lago). Quality of Life measures provide the field with a wide variety of outcome entities that can then be integrated into a profile appropriate to age, disability, functional capacity, and so on.

The reviewers have addressed important elements that require further thought. For example, Lago states that specific domains of QL may be more important during specific time frames of life. Likewise, the potential benefit of a pet may vary in relationship to these times. Observational studies that utilize QL approaches may well be able to assess not only the human but the animal in terms of relationships, benefit, and outcome.

Exception must be taken with selected comments from Marx, who states, "Instruments used in the social sciences are rarely valid or reliable enough to predict specific effects. They are usually intended to suggest very general hypotheses." He raises an interesting point. However, there is a wealth of literature available that supports the strength of various instruments in the health and social sciences that are deemed to have strong reliability and validity (Kane & Kane, 1981; McDowell & Newell, 1987; Spilker, 1990). Our intent in QL research is not to select an instrument on the basis of its "predictive" qualities but rather to select an instrument having strong psychometric characteristics that is also appropriate for the domain we choose to assess.

I appreciate Marx's kind words labeling my previous research as "worthy." However, I urge him to consider that the studies assessing physiologic, psychologic, and social outcomes of pet interaction in college students could well have been conceptualized as part of a quality of life study. QL is now an entity of interest to the National Institutes of Health, especially Heart, Lung, Blood, and Cancer. This "interest" offers HAI researchers the opportunity to piggyback with larger, longitudinal studies, with minimal cost and utilizing existing instruments. Indeed, the anxiety questionnaire used in the research cited by Marx has been used in innumerable studies of hypertension and QL within the past 10 years and is considered to be a strong instrument for assessing for an element of psychological well-being.

These reviewers have conducted well-designed research in the past and, via their own fields, have contributed to the scientific base of human-animal interactions. However, the field itself still suffers from a lack of focus and minimal studies with a sound theoretical and conceptual basis.

Let us look, as epidemiologists purport, "beyond the box" of our own research and utilize specific theoretical/conceptual constructs as a means of evaluating human-animal interactions against accepted "standards." The challenge for HAI research is not whether we can generate well-designed studies dealing with specific subsets of the populations. This has been accomplished. The challenge is whether we can now build a scientific literature that has a unified theory base that allows evaluation of the impact and the process of the human-animal interaction in a wide variety of samples. Thus, we advance the field.

References

Aaronson, N. K. (1989). Quality of life assessment in clinical trials: Methodological issues. *Controlled Clinical Trials, 10,* 195-208S.

Andrews, F. M., & Withey, S. B. (1976). *Social indicators of well-being: The development and measurement of perceptual indicators.* New York: Plenum.

Baun, M. M., Bergstrom, N., Langston, N. F., & Thoma, L. (1984). Psychological effects of human/companion animal bonding. *Nursing Research 3,* 126-129.

Becker, M. H. (Ed.). (1974). *The health belief model and personal health behavior.* Thorofare, NJ: Charles B. Slack.

Bolin, S. E. (1987). The effects of companion animals during conjugal bereavement. *Anthrozoös, 1,* 26-35.

Bradburn, N. (1969). *The structure of psychological well-being.* Chicago: Aldine.

Brickel, C. M., & Brickel, C. K. A. (1980-1981). A review of the role of pet animals on psychotherapy with the elderly. *International Journal on Aging and Human Development, 1*(2), 119-128.

Campbell, A., Converse, P. F., & Rodgers, W. L. (1976). *The quality of American life.* New York: Russell Sage.

Cantril, H. (1965). *Patterns of human concerns.* New Brunswick, NJ: Rutgers University Press.

Colletta, N., & D. Lee. (1983). The impact of support for black adolescent mothers. *Journal of Family Issues, 4,* 127-143.

Connell, C., & Lago, D. J. (1984). Favorable attitudes toward pets and happiness among the elderly. In R. K. Anderson, B. L. Hart, & L. A. Hart (Eds.), *The pet connection: Its influence on our health and quality of life* (pp. 241-250). Minneapolis: University of Minnesota, CENSHARE.

Davis, J. H., & Juhasz, A. M. (1985). The preadolescent/pet bond and psychosocial development. In M. B. Sussman (Ed.), *Pets and the family* (pp. 79-94). New York: Haworth.

DeShriver, M. M., & Riddick, C. C. (1990). Effects of watching aquariums on elders' stress. *Anthrozoös, 4,* 44-48.

Eiseman, B. (1981). The second dimension. *Archives of Surgery, 116,* 11-13.

Feinstein, A. R. (1987). Clinimetric perspectives. *Journal of Chronic Diseases, 40,* 635-640.

Flanagan, J. C. (1978). A research approach to improving our quality of life. *American Psychologist, 33,* 138-147.

88 BEYOND HEALTH

Friedmann, E., Katcher, A. H., Lynch, J. J., & Thomas, S. A. (1980). Animal companions and one year survival of patients after discharge from a coronary care unit. *Public Health Reports, 95,* 307-312.

Friedmann, E., Katcher, A. H., Thomas, S. A., Lynch, J. J., & Messent, P. R. (1983). Social interaction and blood pressure. *Journal of Nervous and Mental Disease, 171,* 461-465.

Friedmann, E., Katcher, A. H., Eaton, M., & Berger, B. (1984). Pet ownership and psychological status. In R. K. Anderson, B. L. Hart, & L. A. Hart (Eds.), *The pet connection: Its influence on our health and quality of life* (pp. 300-308). Minneapolis: University of Minnesota, CENSHARE.

Friedmann, E., & Lockwood, R. (1991). Validation and use of the Animal Thematic Apperception Test (ATAT). *Anthrozoös, 4*(1), 74-83.

Garrity, T. F., Stallones, L., Marx, M. B., & Johnson, T. P. (1989). Pet ownership and attachment as supportive factors in the health of the elderly. *Anthrozoös, 3,* 35-44.

Grossberg, J. M., Alf, F., & Vormbrock, J. K. (1988). Does pet dog presence reduce human cardiovascular responses to stress? *Anthrozoös, 2,* 38-44.

Hollandsworth, I. C. (1988). Evaluating the impact of medical treatment on the quality of life: A 5-year update. *Social Science and Medicine, 26,* 425-434.

Hutchinson, T. A., Boyd, N. F., & Feinstein, A. R. (1979). Scientific problems in clinical scales as demonstrated by the Karnofsky Index of Performance Status. *Journal of Chronic Disease, 32,* 661-666.

Kafer, R, D., Lago, J., Wamboldt, P., & Harrington, F. (1992). The Pet Relationship Scale: Replication of psychometric properties in random samples and association with attitudes toward wild animals. *Anthrozoös, 5,* 93-105.

Kane, R. A., & Kane, R. L. (1981). *Assessing the elderly: A practical guide to measurement.* Lexington, MA: Lexington Books.

Karnofsky, D. A., & Burchenal, J. H. (1949). Clinical evaluation of chemotherapeutic agents in cancer. In C. M. McLeod (Ed.), *Evaluation of chemotherapeutic agents* (pp. 191-205). New York: Columbia University Press.

Katcher, A. H. (1981). Interactions between people and their pets: Form and function. In B. Fogle (Ed.), *Interrelations between people and pets* (pp. 41-67). Springfield, IL: Charles C Thomas.

Lago, D. J., Connell, C. M., & Knight, B. (1985). The effects of animal companionship on older persons living at home. In *Proceedings of the International Symposium on the Occasion of the 80th Birthday of Nobel Prize Winner Professor Dr. Konrad Lorenz* (pp. 34-46). Vienna, Austria: Institute for Interdisciplinary Research on the Human-Pet Relationship.

Lago, D. J., Delaney, M., Miller, M., & Grill, C. (1989). Companion animals, attitudes towards pets and health outcomes among the elderly: A long-term follow-up. *Anthrozoös, 3,* 25-34.

Lago, D. J., Kafer, R., Delaney, M., & Connell, C. (1988). Assessment of favorable attitudes toward pets: Development and preliminary validation of self-report pet relationship scales. *Anthrozoös, 1,* 240-254.

Lago, D. J., Knight, B., & Connell, C. M. (1983). Relationships with companion animals among the rural elderly. In A. H. Katcher & A. M. Beck (Eds.), *New perspectives in our lives with companion animals* (pp. 328-340). Philadelphia: University of Pennsylvania Press.

Levine, M. N., Guyatt, G. H., Gent, M., DePauw, S., Goodyear, M. D., Heyniuk, W. M., Arnold, A., Findlay, B., Skillings, J. R., Bramwell, V. H., Levin, L., Bush, H., Abu-Zahra, H., & Kotalik, J. (1988). Quality of life in slate II breast cancer: An instrument for clinical trials. *Journal of Clinical Oncology 6,* 1798-1810.

McDowell, I., & Newell, C. (1987). *Measuring health: A guide to rating scales and questionnaires.* New York: Oxford University Press.

Marx, M. B. (1984). The salubrious endearment [Review of "New perspectives in our lives with companion animals"]. *Contemporary Psychology, 29,* 902-903.

Melson, G. F. (1990). Studying children's attachment to their pets: A conceptual and methodological review. *Anthrozoös, 4,* 91-99.

Miller, M., & Lago, D. J. (1990a). Observed behavior in pet/owner in-home interactions: Species differences and association with the pet relationship scale. *Anthrozoös, 4,* 49-54.

Miller, M., & Lago, D. J. (1990b). Well-being of older women: The importance of pet and human relations. *Anthrozoös, 3,* 245-252.

Mugford, R. A., & M'Comisky, J. C. (1975). Some recent work on psychotherapeutic value of cage birds with old people. In R. S. Anderson (Ed.), *Pets, animals and society* (pp. 54-65). Baltimore: Williams & Wilkins.

National Institutes of Health. (1988). *Summary of Working Group on Health Benefits of Pets* (DHHS Publication No. 216-107). Washington, DC: Government Printing Office.

Newman, B. M., & Newman, P. R. (1984). *Development through life: A psychosocial approach.* Homewood, IL: Dorsey.

Ory, M. G., & Goldberg, E. L. (1983). Pet possession and well-being in elderly women. *Research on Aging, 5,* 389-409.

Poresky, R. H., Hendrix, C., Mosier, J. E., & Samuelson, M. L. (1987). The companion animal bonding scale: Internal reliability and construct validity. *Psychological Reports, 60,* 743-746.

Rollin, B. E. (1988). Scientism and the human-animal bond. *Anthrozoös, 1,* 150-152.

Rowan, A. N. (1992). The dark side of the force. *Anthrozoös, 5,* 4-5.

Spilker, B. (Ed.). (1990). *Quality of life assessments in clinical trials.* New York: Raven.

Stallones, L., Marx, M. B., Garrity, T. F., & Johnson, T. P. (1990). Pet ownership and attachment in relation to the health of U.S. adults, 21 to 64 years of age. *Anthrozoös, 4,* 100-112.

Unger, D. G., & Powell, D. R. (1980). Supporting families under stress: The role of social networks. *Family Relations, 29,* 566-574.

Wenger, N. K., Mattson, M. I., Furberg, C. D., & Elinson, J. (1984). Overview: Assessment of quality of life in clinical trials of cardiovascular therapies. In N. K. Wenger, M. F. Mattson, C. D. Furberg, & J. Elinson (Eds.), *Assessment of quality of life in clinical trials of cardiovascular therapies* (pp. 1-22). New York: LeJacq.

Wilson, C. C. (1988, September). *Pet ownership and predictive well-being in community based military.* Paper presented at the Seventh Annual Delta Society Meeting, Orlando, FL.

Wilson, C. C. (1991). The pet as an anxiolytic intervention. *Journal of Nervous and Mental Disease, 179,* 482-489.

Wilson, C. C., & Netting, F. E. (1987). New directions: Challenges for human-animal bond research and the elderly. *Journal of Applied Gerontology 7*(2), 51-57.

Wilson, C. C., Netting, F. E., & New, J. C. (1985). Developing the Pet Attitude Inventory: Measuring the human-animal bond. *California Veterinarian, 39*(3), 26-28.

World Health Organization. (1984). *Uses of epidemiology in aging: Report of a scientific group* (Report No. 137). Geneva, Switzerland: Author.

Models for Measuring Quality of Life 5

Implications for Human-Animal
Interaction Research

Ivan Barofsky
Andrew Rowan

Abstract

This chapter reviews basic concepts in Quality of Life Assessment.
It describes the origin of quality of life assessment activities as having originated in a political context serving as an index of the
outcome of various social policy programs. Assessment of Quality
of Life includes measures of happiness and well being. The chapter
also distinguishes between process and outcome measurement in
quality of life assessment. Two basic models of quality of life
assessment are considered; a cognitive model, which takes into
account the fact that the assessment process is an active cognitive
process, and the psychometric perspective which assumed that
while there may be a varition on how people think about quality of
life assessment that this would average out across experimental
conditions. Human-animal bonds occur because much of the impression which forms the basis of happiness and well being may
be produced as much implicitly as explicitly. The role of implicit
learning is therefore discussed as an important mechanism whereby
animals contribute to the well being and satisfaction of humans.

Quality of life (QL) may refer to a variety of frequently overlapping concepts ranging from a measure that can be defined in operational terms and therefore measured (e.g., by the use of an appropriate survey instrument) to a normative concept that is inherently a personal form of moral expression. As a moral concept, it has plagued philosophers from Aristotle (see his discussion of "happiness" in the *Nichomachean Ethics*) to the present. This chapter will initially present selected theoretical issues underlying the definition and measurement of QL. Then suggestions on how the impact of companion animals on quality of life can be assessed and measured are made.

Background

QL assessment is a field as old as humanity because human beings have always reflected on their condition. The formal assessment of quality of life, however, has required that a number of conditions be in place. First, the public has had to convince political representatives that the qualitative aspects of lives was worth assessing. In medicine, practitioners have had to accept that humanistic issues are legitimate concerns that can be incorporated into the practice of medicine. A second major achievement was the demonstration that purely subjective phenomena could be reliably and validly measured, as exemplified by the development of instruments that measured depression or anxiety. Finally, social indicator and health status assessment movements demonstrated that information needed to evaluate and make policy could be made readily available.

Much of the recent interest in QL assessment has evolved from efforts in the early 1960s to establish and evaluate prosocial government programs (Barofsky, 1986). The War on Poverty in the United States is an example of such a program in which quality of life was used as an outcome measure (Campbell, 1981). The idea that programmatic efforts can be evaluated by qualitative outcomes has since expanded to include evaluation of medical interventions. Today, it is fairly common to see QL measures included as part of clinical trials evaluating new medical treatments.

In addition to clinicians, sociologists and economists also became interested in QL and conducted some of the earliest work in the area (Campbell, 1981). In macroeconomics, the gross national product was sometimes viewed as a potential measure of quality of life. Sociologists used indicators such as the poverty rate or people's happiness to determine social progress. The social indicator movement peaked in the 1960s and 1970s but began to wane in response to the technical difficulties of monitoring social change and the political ambivalence toward measuring social processes. Variety of social indicators are still measured in many countries, however (Michalos, 1980).

In its broadest sense, a QL assessment involves clarification of the values held by an individual, a group, or an entire society. QL assessment may be usefully defined as the process of quantifying human values and incorporating them into important human decisions.

Happiness and Satisfaction

Being happy is clearly a valued state. In the United States, the pursuit of happiness is even an element of one of our most significant political documents, the Declaration of Independence. The measurement of happiness, or its surrogate, satisfaction, represents a significant intellectual accomplishment reflecting advances in the assessment of subjective phenomena.

One of the first research observations made in this area was the demonstration that happiness and unhappiness are not opposites (Bradburn, 1969). If a person had many happy feelings, it was not likely that he or she also had many unhappy feelings at the same time (Argyle, 1987). Kammann and Flett (1983) found that the *frequency* of positive and negative feelings were negatively correlated ($r = -.58$). It was possible that a person could have the same *intensity* of feeling, positive or negative, happy or unhappy. A happy person tended to be extroverted, educated, employed, a participant in social and leisure activities, and someone with positive life experiences. In contrast, an unhappy person tended to be neurotic, have low social status and self-esteem, have poor health, and experience stressful life events (Bradburn, 1969; Headey, Holmstrom, & Wearing, 1984; Warr, Barter, & Brownbridge, 1983).

A standard question asked in studies of satisfaction (or happiness) could be phrased as "How satisfied are you with your life as a whole these days?" When this was done in a large national study, it was found that almost 40% of the sample considered themselves nearly but not completely satisfied with their lives. Overall, most people were satisfied with their lives, and few persons admitted being dissatisfied (Campbell, Converse, & Rodgers, 1976).

TABLE 5.1   Sources of Satisfaction in Everyday Life

	Importance	
	Rating, Mean	*Regression Coefficient*
Family life	1.46	0.41
Marriage	1.44	0.36
Financial situation	2.94	0.33
Housing	2.10	0.30
Job	2.19	0.27
Friendship	2.08	0.26
Wealth	1.37	0.22
Leisure activities	2.79	0.21

SOURCE: Angus Campbell, Philip E. Converse, and Willard L. Rodgers, *The Quality of American Life: Perceptions, Evaluations, and Satisfactions.* © 1976 Russell Sage Foundation. Used with permission of Russell Sage Foundation.

Data in Table 5.1 demonstrate that various domains of life contribute different amounts to satisfaction score (Campbell et al., 1976). Thus, financial status is recorded as the most important. As indicated by the regression coefficients, however, family life is mostly highly correlated with a sense of satisfaction. In addition, this hierarchy may change dramatically with varying circumstances, for example, when a person's health declines, leading to health status becoming the most important determinant of satisfaction and dissatisfaction (Argyle, 1987).

Theoretical Issues

QL assessment implies that it is possible to identify a set of rules or operations that will generate the same type of information independent of who is collecting the information. In other words, it assumes that it is possible to operationally define the QL construct. Alternatively, QL can be conceived of as the personal (and essentially private) expression of a person's wants, desires, and interests. If one assumes that quality of life is rooted in individual wants, then defending the autonomy of individuals so that they can define their own concepts of the good life is a form of moral expression (Faden & LePlege, 1992). In such circumstances, can any formal assessment take into account individual uniqueness but still permit general statements? This question constantly plagues efforts to measure QL. Empirically, however, sufficient commonality is found between individuals to provide a basis for measurement.

Distinguishing Process and Outcome in QL Measurement

The difference between process and outcome is an important distinction in QL assessment. General consensus is that a QL assessment is an outcome measure (Barofsky, 1996; Patrick & Erickson, 1993). Many psychosocial variables, however, are presumed to measure QL but are better understood as process variables. It is not uncommon to read in the literature that a person in pain or who is depressed has a poor quality of life. If a person is in pain or is depressed and these feelings affect the ability of the person to function, then the change in functioning is a QL measure. In contrast, the coping activities that the same person engages in to deal with pain or depression are psychosocial or process measures.

This distinction is not a trivial one, as shown in a discussion of the results of research that tried to determine if women who received a lumpectomy or total mastectomy had a better quality of life (Barofsky, 1996). Typically, the literature has been interpreted as indicating that there was no difference in QL as a function of the type of breast surgery when only 2 of the 19 studies included a standardized QL assessment, and 3 included a clinically developed QL assessment. All other studies included one or more psychosocial assessments, assessments that measured coping style, attribution, social support, emotional distress, denial, and so on. From these data, the consistent observation was that patients who had a total mastectomy suffered from altered body images. Using the process-outcome distinction, the observed body image change would be considered a process measure, and the empirical question is to determine if the body image change led to an outcome change, such as reduced frequency of putting on swimsuits, increased avoidance of being naked in front of husbands, reduced frequency of intimate encounters, and so on. Thus, the failure to distinguish between process and outcome measures in the mastectomy studies leaves unanswered the question of who enjoys a better quality of life—a woman who has had a lumpectomy or a woman who has had a total mastectomy.

In the human-animal bond literature, relatively few attempts have been made to measure the impact of pet ownership on QL. Generally, it has been

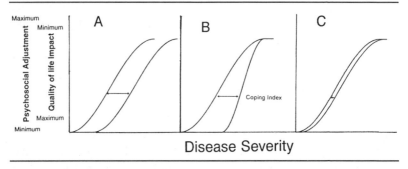

Disease Severity

Figure 5.1. The Relationship Between Psychosocial Adjustment and Quality of Life
SOURCE: From *Quality of Life and Pharmacoeconomics in Clinical Trials* (p. 996), by B. Spilker (Ed.), 1996, New York: Raven. Copyright © 1996 by Lippincott-Raven Publishers. Reprinted with permission.
NOTE: Plotted in the figure are three models of the relationship between psychosocial adjustment and quality of life impact. The basic relationship depicted is that as disease severity increases, the capacity of an individual to adapt psychologically decreases and the impact of the disease increases. Also implied in each panel is that quality of life impact (right-hand function) will be delayed relative to psychosocial change.

accepted that pet ownership has a cardioprotective effect (Rowan & Beck, 1994) and reduces anxiety (Wilson, 1991). Using the distinction between outcome and process, proving that pet ownership would favorably affect QL requires the demonstration that owning a pet leads to changed function, a change that the person values. Thus, reduced anxiety that comes from pet ownership (a process measure) would affect QL only if this reduced anxiety led to increased valued function.

Figure 5.1 graphically illustrates the distinction between psychosocial (process) and QL (outcome) measures. It is assumed that psychosocial and QL measures are dose sensitive and will change as disease severity (the dose) increases. As the disease progresses, the individual's capacity to adjust reaches a peak and then levels off. The adverse impact on QL may increase but then also reaches a peak and levels off. The two processes may not be parallel, and a person's capacity to adjust may vary without any significant impact on the QL. For example, depressed persons actively cope with their depression and yet continue to function well enough to hide their distress—distress that remains unrevealed until a chance event or question reveals its extent.

The distance between the two functions, located at the midpoint of change, was defined as a measure of overall coping. This "coping index" is analogous to the therapeutic index, which refers to the difference between the drug dose that is effective in treating a disease compared with a dose that causes severe side effects. The larger the therapeutic index, the safer the drug. The coping index measures the person's adjustment capacity (i.e., reflecting a person's capacity to cope, deny, etc.) and the ability to forestall QL changes. The larger the coping index, the more likely people can live with a particular situation without it disrupting their life quality.

The coping index could be a useful method of measuring the value of companion animals. For example, it might be possible to demonstrate that companion animals help persons deal with life stressors better, which should then be reflected as an increase in the coping index. An increase in the coping index would mean that the distance between the psychosocial adjustment and QL functions would be increased (Figure 5.1). Allen and Blascovich (1996) report that the acquisition of a service dog by persons with severe ambulatory difficulties improves a variety of psychosocial adjustments (i.e., as measured by changes in self-esteem, internal locus of control, psychological well-being, and community integration), which might then be reflected in the person's level of functioning or QL.

Types of Outcome Measures: Reference Groups

If QL assessment is an outcome measure, then it is evident that there are several ways of measuring outcome, each differing in the reference group being assessed. First, in some approaches to measuring QL, the investigator may attempt to characterize the "good" life. This approach implies that there is a philosophical ideal and that this ideal can be measured and reached. An individual, clinician, or policymaker may consider an ideal goal to be impractical. Thus, an alternative approach is to define the goal as what is true for the population as a whole. For example, if one sought to ensure a certain sense of personal security, one would have to develop a suitable measure of personal security and then evaluate how the presence of companion animals might increase feelings of personal security to a desirable level.

It may not be practical to define the outcome of an activity in the population as a whole. Instead, it may be necessary to select a specific group and use characteristics of the specific group to evaluate a particular intervention. An example is the study of Allen and Blascovich (1996), in which the impact of a companion animal on a select group of individuals who were severely restricted in their ability to move around was evaluated.

Models of Quality of Life Assessment

♥♥ A QL assessment is an activity in which people ordinarily engage.
♥♥ What a person does, however, can be described in different ways. For example, a person can select and combine specific experiences, estimate the intensity of these experiences, indicate a preference for these experiences, and aggregate these experiences into some composite "impression." It is this impression that a person would provide if asked to indicate his or her QL. This approach to QL suggests that the person is engaging in an active thought process. The understanding of this thought process provides insight into the nature of a QL assessment. These activities are referred to as a cognitive model of QL.

Cognitive Models

Historically, the cognitive model of QL assessment has evolved from two traditions (i.e., psychology and economics). Both are involved with studies of decision making and judgment. The decision-making model, for example, assumes that humans can make rational decisions and ordinarily do things to maximize their gains and minimize their losses. This "rational human" model has been used as a justification for developing scales that measure health-related QL such that perfect health is scored as a one and death is scored as zero. This model has been used to assess individual preferences, and such data have been used to set policy (Kaplan, 1993).

Norman Anderson's (1991) "cognitive algebra" or "information integration" theory evolved from psychophysics and attempts to account for how information is used. Anderson assumes that people use various algebraic techniques to manage the information they receive and then to make choices based on that information. Veit, Rose, and Ware (1982) report a study that evaluated this model and in which respondents were asked to indicate their preference for combinations of physical and mental health states. Preferences were determined by a questionnaire that was based on a factorial design resulting in 256 comparisons (all possible combinations). Each health state was ranked at five levels. Results revealed that the functions that were generated were parallel, suggesting that the way people make comparisons follows an additive model. If these functions had been nonparallel, it would suggest an interaction, or that people combine information in a multiplicative manner.

Social judgment theory has been used to generate a procedure whereby it is possible to measure an individual's QL and is based on Egon Bruniswik's ecological approach to psychology (Hammond, McClelland, & Mumpower, 1980). The model involves externalizing a person's thought processes (McGee, O'Boyle, Hickey, O'Malley, & Joyce, 1991). Persons are first asked to list the five most important areas of life that contribute to their QL. They are then asked to rate each area as how good or how bad things are for them. They are also asked to provide an overall judgment of their QL. The next stage is to ask them to consider different theoretical combinations of outcomes for the five areas of most interest and to generate an overall judgment. From this, it is possible to understand how persons' valuation of the individual domains correlates with their overall judgment of QL. Data suggest that this method is capable of describing different patterns of outcome as a function of the health state of the individual (Browne et al., 1994). Most important, this work has evolved from a theoretical model of cognitive processes. By so doing, it avoids the arbitrariness of psychometric approaches.

John Anderson's (1993) ACT-R theory has not, as yet, found application in QL assessment. Based on information processing theory, this theory approaches directly the issues of unconscious cognitive events and the role they may play in QL assessment. This theory is based on memory and how memory works (Kihlstrom, 1987). A central tenet is that although humans may be aware of our goals and the status of our activities, we are not aware of the operations leading to these outcomes. This forms a logic basis for understanding the role of companion animals in determining QL.

An animal becomes a part of our life as a result of our learning about it and experiencing its behavior and needs. Increasingly clear, however, is that we may be aware of only part of what we learn from interacting with an animal and that there may be a part that we learn implicitly (Reber, 1993).

Because we are not aware of this implicit learning, special efforts may be necessary to demonstrate that it has occurred. For example, we learn grammar implicitly, and unless specifically taught, most people could not describe and explain the grammatical rules they follow in everyday speech.

It is possible that living with animals teaches humans something that fits this category of learning. We may learn self-confidence, control over the world, and enhanced self-esteem as a result of the process of dealing with animals. This all may occur at a unconscious level. The study of this phenomenon and how it contributes to QL assessment is a promising research topic.

Psychometric Models

An alternative but more common approach evolves from the reality that a person's QL is based on many experiences and that any assessment instrument inevitably samples a limited portion of these experiences. As a result, the assessment instrument has to be characterized by the degree it represents the broad array of possible experiences (i.e., its representativeness). In addition, the sample of items on the questionnaire must capture what the test is meant to measure. It is also necessary to determine if the selected sample of items can reliably describe the construct being evaluated, which in this case is QL. The entire field involved in establishing the characteristics of an assessment instrument is called psychometrics. The psychometric approach has been successful in generating a host of assessment instruments to measure QL (e.g., Spilker, 1996).

Conclusion

This chapter has introduced the richness and complexity of QL assessment as it relates to human-animal interactions. It is one of the few intellectual activities that affords the opportunity to consider philosophic and biologic elements in the same context. It raises ethical, measurement, and policy issues.

Companion animals can fit into such QL assessments in several ways. It is specifically suggested that one of these ways is that the impact of animals is acquired implicitly and expressed implicitly. If this is the case, then new assessment methods may have to be applied before the role of animals in QL is to be fairly evaluated.

References

Allen, K., & Blascovich, J. (1996). The value of service dogs for people with severe ambulatory difficulties. *Journal of the American Medical Association, 275,* 1001-1006.

Anderson, J. R. (1993). *Rules of the mind.* Hillsdale, NJ: Lawrence Erlbaum.

Anderson, N. H. (1991). *Contributions to information integration theory* (Vols. 1-3). Hillsdale, NJ: Lawrence Erlbaum.

Argyle, M. (1987). *The psychology of happiness.* London: Routledge.

Barofsky, I. (1986). Quality of life assessment: Evolution of a concept. In V. Ventaffrida, R. Yancik, F. S. A. M. van Dam, & M. Tamburini (Eds.), *Quality of life assessment and cancer treatment* (pp. 11-18). Amsterdam: Elsevier.

Barofsky, I. (1996). Cognitive aspects of quality of life assessment. In B. Spilker (Ed.), *Quality of life and pharmacoeconomics in clinical trials* (2nd ed., pp. 107-115). New York: Raven.

Bradburn, N. M. (1969). *The structure of psychological well-being.* Chicago: Aldine.

Browne, J. P., O'Boyle, C. A., McGee, H. M., Joyce, C. R. B., McDonald, N. J., O'Malley, K., & Hiltbrunner, B. (1994). Individual quality of life in the healthy elderly. *Quality of Life Research, 3,* 235-244.

Campbell, A. (1981). *The sense of well-being in America.* New York: McGraw-Hill.

Campbell, A., Converse, P. E., Rodgers, W. L. (1976). *The quality of American life.* New York: Russell Sage.

Faden, R., & LePlege, A. (1992). Assessing quality of life: Moral implications for clinical practice. *Medical Care, 30*(Suppl. 5), 166-175.

Hammond, K. R., McClelland, G. H., & Mumpower, J. (1980). *Human judgment and decision making: Theories, methods and procedures.* New York: Praeger.

Headey, B., Holmstrom, E., & Wearing A. (1984). Well-being and ill-being: Different dimensions? *Social Indicators Research, 14,* 115-139.

Kammann, R., & Flett, R. (1983). Affectometer 2: A scale to measure current level of general happiness. *Australian Journal of Psychology, 35,* 259-265.

Kaplan, R. M. (1993). *Hippocratic predicament: Affordability, access and accountability in health care.* San Diego, CA: Academic Press.

Kihlstrom, J. F. (1987). The cognitive unconscious. *Science, 237,* 1445-1452.

McGee, H. M., O'Boyle, C. A., Hickey, A., O'Malley, K., & Joyce, C. R. B. (1991). Assessing the quality of life of the individual: The SEOQL with a healthy and a gastroenterology unit population. *Psychological Medicine, 21,* 749-759.

Michalos, A. C. (1980). *North American social report: A comparative study of the quality of life in Canada and the USA from 1964 to 1974.* Dordrecht, The Netherlands: Reidel.

Patrick, D. L., & Erickson, P. (1993). *Health status and health policy: Quality of life and health care evaluation and resource allocation.* New York: Oxford University Press.

Reber, A. S. (1993). *Implicit learning and tact knowledge: An essay on the cognitive unconscious.* New York: Oxford University Press.

Rowan, A. N., & Beck, A. M. (1994). The health benefits of human-animal interactions. *Anthrozoös, 7,* 85-89.

Spilker, B. (Ed.). (1996). *Quality of life and pharmacoeconomics in clinical trials.* New York: Raven.

Veit, C. T., Rose, B. J., & Ware, J. E. (1982). Effects of physical and mental health on health state preferences. *Medical Care, 20,* 386-401.

Warr, P., Barter, J., & Brownbridge, G. (1983). On the independence of positive and negative affect. *Journal of Personality and Social Psychology, 44,* 644-651.

Wilson, C. C. (1991). The pet as an anxiolytic intervention. *Journal of Nervous and Mental Disease, 172,* 482-489.

PART III

Quality of Life Outcomes: Psychosocial Aspects of Human-Animal Interactions

Cindy C. Wilson
Dennis C. Turner

Variables from two domains of QL (i.e., psychological and sociological) are frequently assessed as outcome markers in QL and HAI studies. In this segment, Collis and McNicholas propose a theoretical basis for health benefits (i.e., QL benefits) by determining whether attachment or social support offers the best means of explaining positive QL outcomes. Also in this context, Keil examines the relationship of attachment, loneliness, and stress in older adults. Her findings in a fairly select sample echo data previously reported (Ory & Goldberg, 1984), which found that older women living in nonrural communities who had close confidants aside from their spouses were most likely to have a pet and report higher levels of happiness. As Barofsky and Rowan suggested in the previous section, happiness, a valued QL factor, attachment, and the reference group assessed may be interrelated. Clearly, the depth and breadth of social support available is emerging as an important variable from all these studies. Triebenbacher combines components from attachment and self-esteem theory and applies them to young children, finding that elements of Cobb's social support theory emerge. The unconditional love, commitment between child and animal, and the sense of self-esteem engendered are consistent with positive QL outcomes from human-animal interactions.

Reference

Ory, M. G., & Goldberg, E. L. (1984). An epidemiological study of pet ownership. In R. K. Anderson, B. L. Hart, & L. A. Hart (Eds.), *The pet connection* (pp. 320-330). Minneapolis: University of Minnesota, CENSHARE.

A Theoretical Basis for Health Benefits of Pet Ownership 6

Attachment Versus Psychological Support

Glyn M. Collis
June McNicholas

Abstract

A number of studies suggest an association between pet ownership and advantages for health, but the underlying processes are not clear. One hypothesis is that the relationship between person and pet could directly influence the owner's health. This motivates exploration of issues concerning the nature and function(s) of these relationships. These relationships are most likely based on psychological mechanisms other than attachment or other motivationally driven mechanisms that underlie human-human relationships but not specifically attachment relationships. Despite its attraction as an intriguing issue that should yield to scientific analysis, the nature of person-pet relationships is still not well understood. The hypothesis that they mediate associations between pet ownership and advantages for physical health and psychological well-being gives a sharper focus to research on these relationships.

AUTHORS' NOTE: During the preparation of this chapter, we received financial support from the Waltham Centre for Pet Nutrition. June McNicholas is a Waltham Research Fellow.

Numerous reports in the last 20 years have suggested that pet ownership is associated with health advantages (e.g., Anderson, Reid, & Jennings, 1992; Friedmann, Katcher, Lynch, & Thomas, 1980; Mugford & M'Comisky, 1975; Serpell, 1991; Siegel, 1990). The result has been a widespread acceptance of a causal connection between pet ownership and health. Despite a few critical commentaries (Wright & Moore, 1982), the literature overall seems noncritical in its acceptance of the causal hypothesis.

It is important to replicate and extend studies supporting an association between pet ownership and health advantages, yet such studies should be complemented by investigations of the mechanisms underlying the associations. There are three broad classes of explanation for associations between pet ownership and health, the most obvious is that pets have a direct causal effect on human health. The alternatives are (a) that pet ownership has an indirect effect on health by facilitating person-to-person relations and (b) that other factors influence both pet ownership and health but that pet ownership has no causal effect on health. We further discuss the latter two alternatives in Chapter 11.

One hypothesis for a direct causal effect is that health advantages are a consequence of the relationship between the person and the pet. A second hypothesis is that there are direct effects at a physiological level, for example, the presence of a pet moderates cardiovascular responses such as blood pressure changes (Friedmann, 1995). Direct physiological effects could, but need not, occur within the context of a person-pet relationship (as opposed to a short-term acquaintance with the particular animal).

Effects of Person-Pet Relationships on Health: A Guiding Assumption

It is useful to define an assumption that is implicit in many references to social relationships in the literature on companion animals. This assumption is not original, but by clarifying an idea that underlies much contemporary thinking, it can be critically evaluated and alternatives can be clearly recognized. We phrase the assumption as follows:

It is unlikely that the human species has evolved or otherwise acquired a set of psychological processes whose primary function is to serve relationships with companion animals; it is much more likely that these processes are "borrowed" from those used in human-human relationships and used for human-animal relationships.

It is not anti-Darwinian or anti-ethological to prefer this position to the alternative view that *Homo sapiens* has evolved some distinct processes for interacting or relating to companion animals (cf. Herzog & Burghardt, 1987; Serpell, 1987). It is entirely consistent with evolutionary theory to envisage "old" structures or processes being applied in new contexts. New functions may provide an impetus for further evolutionary change, as when feathers were "discovered" to have useful aerodynamic properties, but further adaptation is not a necessary consequence of such a situation.

There are two significant corollaries to the assumption. First, concepts used in the study of human relationships, including attachment, social support, and many others, are considerably more than metaphors in helping to understand humans' relationships with companion animals; they can be explored and accepted or rejected as they stand. Second, discoveries made about human-companion animal relationships may reveal new insights into the nature of human-human relationships.

Categories and Functions of Social Relationships

One way to use the assumption to aid the inquiry into person-pet relationships is to ask whether a particular category of person-person relationships will help explain the characteristics of person-pet relationships. The classic categories of relationships are child-to-parent attachment relationships, parent-to-child caregiving relationships, child-to-child peer relationships, and adult-to-adult sexual relationships. It has been suggested that these have distinct psychobiological substrates (Harlow & Harlow, 1965). Other types of relationships could be added to this list, perhaps most important, sibling relationships and adult friendships. If person-pet relationships were to fit anywhere on this list, the literature on companion animals suggests attachment as the prime candidate, perhaps with parent-to-child caregiving as a second possibility.

An alternative to focusing on categories of relationship is to focus directly on the functional mechanisms by which relationships might promote advantages for health. A functional approach need not be constrained by descriptive categories of relationships. A natural way to follow this strategy is to examine the supportive functions of relationships. Social or psychological support has emerged specifically as an explanation of variations in health and disease. Concepts of support also feature in the literature on companion animals (McNicholas & Collis, 1995).

Bonds and Attachments

In the literature on companion animals, pet-person relationships are most commonly characterized as bonds or attachments, but it is not always clear how these terms are used. In its narrow technical meaning, an attachment refers to the close relationship, based on feelings of security, of a young child to a parent (Bowlby, 1969). A slightly broader technical use could encompass other relationships known to be derived from child-parent attachments or based on the same narrowly defined psychobiological mechanisms, particularly felt security (Ainsworth, 1989). What is meant by security in this context is important and is discussed in the next section. The concept of a bond, even in its technical use, is considerably broader than attachment. A bond is the affection and attraction felt by one individual for another "particular individual"—not for a group or a species (Bowlby, 1979). In this framework, the meaning of bond is broadly similar to what most people think of as a close relationship. It is unfortunate that the term *bond* is sometimes used broadly, as in "the human-animal bond." More confusion has probably been caused by the lay use of *attachment* to denote almost any type of close relationship.

The concepts of attachment and bonding, as developed in ethology and psychology, are primarily concerned with child-parent relationships. One of the most striking features of child-parent relationships is the asymmetry between the thinking and language skills of the adult and the relative lack of sophistication of these skills in the child. It might therefore seem attractive to apply these concepts to person-pet relationships, which are also asymmetrical. The similarity, however, is more apparent than real. The classic formulation of attachment (Bowlby, 1969) is about psychological benefits accruing to the less cognitively sophisticated individual, the child, who is attached to the parent. In person-pet relationships, the asymmetry is the other way around. The cognitively sophisticated person is seen as attached to the less sophisticated animal, with psychological benefits accruing to the person.

A superficially similar theoretical framework was developed to cover the so-called bonding of a parent to the child (Klaus & Kennell, 1976). In this framework, there was a brief critical period for the formation of the bond, a process based on rapid learning quite unlike the gradual emergence of a child's attachment to a parent. In most other respects, it is quite unlike child-to-parent attachment. Although the parent-child relationship is an important and perhaps archetypal example of a relationship based on caregiving (Ainsworth, 1989), many of the main conclusions from Klaus and Kennell's work are now seen to be erroneous in many respects (Myers, 1984; Sluckin, Herbert, & Sluckin, 1983).

Attachment Theory

To examine the case that person-pet relationships are like attachments, it is necessary to look more deeply into attachment theory and to examine ways in which it has been extended into the domain of adult-adult human relationships where the role of the two individuals is more symmetrical, which is unlike child-to-parent attachment, parent-to-child caregiving relationships, or person-pet relationships.

Two principles were fundamental to Bowlby's (1969) original ideas on the mechanisms of attachment. These principles have played a key role in subsequent research by Bowlby and others.

Principle 1: Attachment as a Motivational System

Child-to-parent attachment behavior was postulated to be controlled by a biologically based motivational system. A key feature of the attachment system was that presence of the attachment figure (typically the mother) enhanced felt security. A lack of felt security (felt insecurity), which might arise in a broad variety of circumstances, triggered the production of attachment behavior with the goal of reestablishing proximity, much the same way as feelings of hunger might be said to trigger feeding. The role of felt security/insecurity in this system was not assumed to depend on, or derive from, the child's experiencing the removal of sources of insecurity, anxiety, or alarm by the attachment figure. Nor was the role dependent on the child's understanding that the attachment figure could remove a source of threat. The attachment system was seen as a primary motive produced by evolutionary design with the function of ensuring the protection and safety of the child without the child having the cognitive capability to comprehend the nature of danger, except in the most rudimentary way of feeling insecure (e.g., unfamiliar surroundings and in the absence of the mother).

It is not proximity seeking that defines the attachment motivational system. Sexual motivation also involves proximity seeking. The key elements are the role of felt insecurity as the motivational force behind proximity seeking and the development of the motivational system without specific experience (although specific experience is involved in selecting the attachment figure).

Bowlby (1969) distinguished the attachment system from a number of other affectional systems such as the parent-to-child caregiving system, the adult-to-adult sexual system, and the peer friendship system (Harlow & Harlow, 1965). Bowlby's concept of an affectional system is based on the concept of motivational system in ethology (e.g., Hinde, 1966). The assumption that distinct motivational systems serve different types of relationships underpins the idea that there are natural categories of relationships. Most major attempts to characterize adult human relationships through attachment theory identify a key role for motivation based on felt security/insecurity (e.g., Ainsworth, 1989; Weiss, 1982; West & Sheldon-Keller, 1994).

Principle 2: Internal Working Models

Although Bowlby (1969) borrowed the concept of motivational system from ethology, he borrowed the concept of a mental model from cognitive psychology. Bowlby argued that on the basis of the first attachment, the young child begins to organize experiences and expectations of social interactions into internal working models of the self, of the attachment figure, and, in effect, of the attachment relationship. An internal working model is a system of cognitive representations that works as a knowledge base. Bowlby argued that working models of the attachment relationship form the basis of mental models of other affectional relationships that develop subsequently. In this way, cognitive representations of the first relationship could influence various relationships in adult life. There are different views, however, on the nature of this influence. The influence might be relatively minor, with early models subject to extensive modification by subsequent experiences (Bretherton, 1985, 1987). The influence might be rather profound, particularly in the way that feelings of security/insecurity feature in the model and influence social behavior and relationships of various types in adulthood (e.g., Main, Caplan, & Cassidy, 1985).

The Scope of Attachment Theory

The last decade has seen a marked upsurge of interest in characterizing adult relationships through attachment theory, particularly since Hazan & Shaver (1987) argued that many romantic relationships are essentially attachments (see also Sperling & Berman, 1994). The enthusiasm for the idea of adult attachments has highlighted the importance of carefully considering the boundaries of the concept of attachment. If the concept is made too general, it will lose explanatory power and end up explaining nothing. This concern seems to have led to a series of articles from Mary Ainsworth (especially 1989). A major attachment theorist who worked alongside Bowlby in the early years in the development of the theory, Ainsworth has been the most important single influence on its subsequent development. She has clarified the issue of what is an attachment relationship in the conceptual scheme depicted in Figure 6.1. Ainsworth suggests that a subset of adult human relationships are properly regarded as affectional bonds if based on a long-enduring tie in which the partner is important as a unique individual. The key psychological process underlying the tie is an internal working model of the relationship. The tie may be maintained during absences, but there is a desire to come together and pleasure in doing so. Because there are affectional aspects to the tie, separation will cause distress, and loss will cause grief.

Some, but not all, affectional bonds are attachments. An important criterion of an attachment is the reduction of felt insecurity in the presence of the partner, which is presumed to be a consequence of the activation of motivational system. An alternative interpretation is that early in life, the operation of the attachment motivational system so influenced cognitive models of relationships that the style of responding to felt insecurity is a major dimension of individual differences in social relationships. Ainsworth explicitly indicates that a mother's bond to her child is not properly called an attachment because felt security is typically not a major feature of this type of bond. In a recent article on parents' cognitive working models, George (1996) describes distinct patterns of representations for caregiving and attachment.

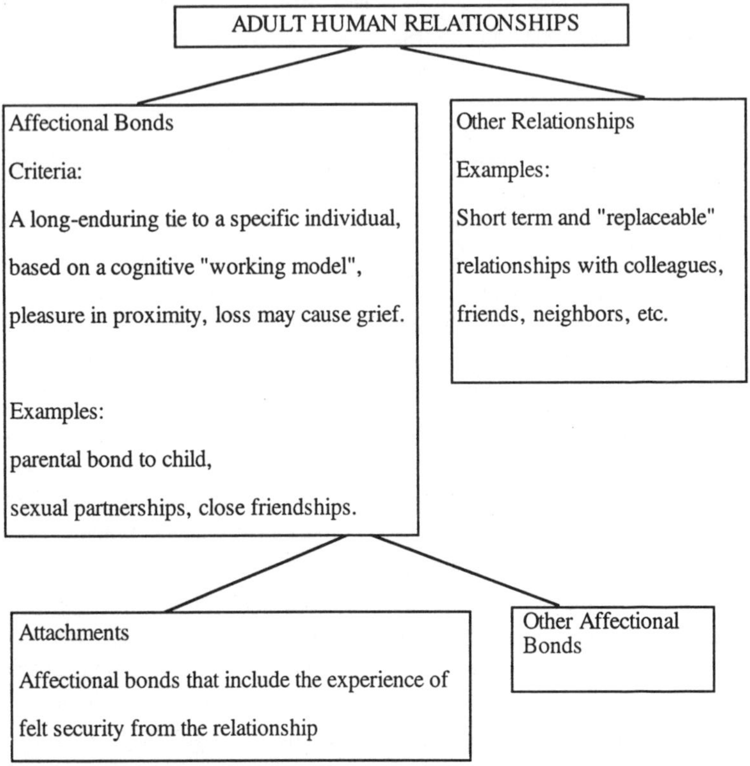

Figure 6.1. Ainsworth's Typology for Adult Human Relationships From the Perspective of Attachment Theory

Any affectional bond may have components from different affectional systems. For example, marital relationships typically involve sexual attraction, caring for offspring, caring for the partner, and experiencing comfort and security from the presence of the partner. Only if the last component is present is such a relationship properly called an attachment. West and Sheldon-Keller (1994) take this approach further by suggesting that "any relationship may have an attachment component to the degree that the relationship promotes security. A relationship becomes an attachment relationship when the primary purpose of the relationship is the provision of security" (p. 160).

Person-Pet Relationships as Attachments

It is unlikely that felt security is particularly important in most person-pet relationships. In evaluating this claim, it is important to distinguish between felt security in the rather nonspecific affective sense used to define the attachment motivational system and a more focused cognitive appraisal of a specific role (e.g., a large dog in acting as a deterrent or defender against mugging or burglary). The type of insecurity that plays a central role in Bowlby's theory is a primary motivation, which will initiate proximity seeking regardless of whether the child has had the opportunity to learn that the attachment figure could remove specific threats.

To date, attempts to quantify people's relationships with pets have not tapped feelings or attitudes that relate closely to attachment theory. As examples, the CENSHARE Pet Attachment Survey (Holcombe, Williams, & Richards, 1985), the Lexington Attachment to Pets Scale (Johnson, Garrity, & Stallones, 1991), and the Companion Animal Bonding Scale (Poresky, Hendrix, Mosier, & Samuelson, 1987) contain items that loosely reflect the desire for proximity with a pet (especially sleeping with or near the pet), but there is little else related to attachment theory. In contrast, most methods for assessing attachment in adult relationships lead to classifications or measurements based on security (Crowell & Treboux, 1995). Moreover, little attempt has been made to compare items that should reflect attachment-like relationships with items that reflect social relationships of other types. Although scales are routinely subjected to factor analysis to see whether different dimensions can be identified, inspection of the eigenvalues (i.e., percentage of variance explained by each factor) strongly suggests that these scales each represent only a single dimension. Although multidimensional structures are often reported, there seems to have been undue reliance on the default setting used by standard statistical packages that imply that eigenvalues greater than 1.0 indicate a distinct dimension, a criterion known to be misleading (Zwick & Velicer, 1986). The nature of the items suggests that the main dimension resembles a measure of generalized close and affectionate relationships rather than attachment.

Feelings of great sadness at the loss of a pet are often interpreted as grief, an interpretation that has been used to strengthen the concept that the person-pet relationship is like attachment (Archer & Winchester, 1993;

Rajaram, Garrity, Stallones, & Marx, 1993). Conceptually, in Ainsworth's scheme, grief is a characteristic of affectional bonds in general, rather than attachment in particular. Empirically, responses to pet loss are varied, and even when marked, they are seldom as long-lasting, as intense, or as disruptive as those experienced following the loss of a close human relationship (McNicholas & Collis, 1995).

The attachment metaphor is not helpful in characterizing human-animal relationships that are presumed to borrow from a pool of motivational and cognitive components, strategies, and dispositions available in human-human relationships. Attachment mechanisms may have contributed to this pool but do not explain the implications of pet ownership. It is not particularly helpful to focus on attachment, rather than on any other category of relationships. A promising alternative is to focus on what person-pet relationships do for people and how they might work to influence health.

Supportive Functions of Person-Pet Relationships

The process-oriented concept of *support* is particularly attractive as a framework for understanding how person-pet relationships produce health advantages. This framework is not new to the field (Friedmann et al., 1980), but the ways in which it differs from other approaches have not been well studied. The concept of support emerged specifically as a framework for understanding the effects of social and psychological factors on health and well-being across the life span, contrasting with the roots of attachment theory in developmental psychology and psychopathology. Moreover, there need be no a priori assumptions about the motivational underpinnings or developmental histories of relationships that provide support. Many types of relationships can be supportive on the basis of what they do for people. It has been argued that theories of supportive and attachment relationships have much in common (Sarason, Pierce, & Sarason, 1990). Yet neither the theory nor the evidence for this is particularly strong. Considering the difficulties in accommodating person-pet relationships within the concept of attachment, that approach seems inappropriate in the present context.

Social support is an omnibus term covering a variety of acts or interpersonal transactions in social relationships. An early conceptualization of social support was that of Cobb (1976), who described it as information leading to one or more of three outcomes: feelings of being cared for; the belief that one is loved, esteemed, and valued; and the sense of belonging to a reciprocal network. Cobb believed that social support provided protection from pathological states and accelerated recovery from illnesses by acting as a buffer in times of crisis. Although a number of multidimensional models of social support have been proposed by theorists and researchers, few have strayed far from Cobb's original conceptualization, and their ideas about the different forms or components of social support appear to converge on a common set of dimensions. Most commonly cited are the following:

1. Emotional support: the ability to turn to others for comfort in times of stress, leading the person to feel cared for by others
2. Social integration or network support: the feeling of being a part of a group with common interests and concerns (this may range from close relationships such as within a family, to work relationships or casual friendships that enable social and recreational activities)
3. Esteem support: the bolstering of a person's sense of competence and self-worth, value to others, respect, and self-respect (e.g., giving positive feedback regarding a person's abilities or worth)
4. Tangible/practical/instrumental support: the giving of concrete assistance or resources (e.g., the provision of physical help with a task and lending money at a time of financial difficulty)
5. Informational support: the giving of advice or guidance
6. Opportunity to provide nurturance: the need to be needed

Companionship is seen as theoretically distinct from social support (Rook, 1990) in that it does not offer extrinsic support but provides intrinsic satisfactions such as shared pleasure in recreation, relaxation, and uncensored spontaneity. Companionship may be important in fostering positive mental health, whereas social support may be more important in buffering threats to mental health from stressors.

Major stressful life events have been shown repeatedly to increase the incidence of adverse physical and/or psychological responses, resulting in illness, depression, and so on. There is considerable evidence that social support may alleviate such reactions and be an important source of variability in how people respond to stress. Support may also accelerate recovery from illness, even serious medical conditions such as stroke (Glass, Matchar, Belyea, & Feussner, 1993), myocardial infarction (Fontana, Kerns, Rosenberg, & Colonese, 1989; Kulik & Mahler, 1993), and cancer

(Wortman, 1984). Absence of social support, feelings of isolation, and actual loneliness exacerbate existing stresses and predispose to further stresses.

At least two factors influence the effectiveness of support in reducing stress. The first is whether the act or information is perceived to be supportive by the recipient, regardless of how supportive or well-intentioned it is perceived to be by the provider or others outside the transaction. Similarly, provided that the recipient regards an act as supportive, it is unimportant whether the actor or others outside the transaction agree or not.

Second, to be effective, the type of support must match the specific needs of the recipient at the time (Cutrona & Russell, 1990). If someone really needs comfort (emotional support) or reassurance of his or her capabilities (esteem support) after failing an exam, it is of little use to offer advice on alternative careers (informational support) or a lift to the social security office (practical support). At some later stage, both of these may be regarded as supportive by the recipient, but not at the earlier stage when the recipient is still pained by experience. Support that is ill-matched to a need may be particularly damaging by undermining the recipient's confidence in a relationship. Similarly, inconsistent support can be anxiety provoking. Yet it is common for burnout to occur in providers of social support, resulting in gradually diminishing support, or fluctuations in support, regardless of the actual need of the recipient.

Support in Person-Pet Relationships

Some types of social support feature strongly in person-pet relationships and are candidates for a causal role in the health advantages seen among pet owners. The term *candidates* is stressed because most of the evidence to date is descriptive and anecdotal. High-quality empirical research is required to establish whether concepts of support really have explanatory power when applied to person-pet relationships.

Descriptions of pet ownership often feature emotional and esteem support as elements of the relationship. It is plausible that these aspects of perceived support from a pet may have greater stability than similar elements of support from a human relationship. That pets are not human may be advantageous because there is no fear that the relationship will be damaged by displays of weakness, emotion, or by excessive demands.

The opportunity to provide nurturance was suggested as a form of support by Weiss (1974). Because it could be seen as increasing one's sense of competence or worth, it might also be considered a form of esteem support. The opportunity to provide nurturance is particularly relevant for person-pet relationships. In certain circumstances, pets may provide instrumental support, (e.g., service animals such as guide dogs and assistance dogs). Network support may be provided or enhanced by pets through their role as social catalysts enhancing person-person contacts (McNicholas, Collis, Morley, & Lane, 1993; Messent, 1983). If this enhanced their owners' network of human relationships and these human relationships conveyed health advantages for the owners, this would be a case of an indirect causal effect of pets on health (see Chapter 11), whereas other types of support from pets are more likely to produce direct effects.

It is established that sources and effectiveness of support may become discernible only at times of stress. If support is derived from pets, the benefits would be expected to become apparent only during stress, when such support may relieve stress or act as a buffer against adverse health effects (Cohen & Wills, 1985). It is therefore predictable that investigations of target populations undergoing some adverse life event should be most likely to detect effects of pet ownership. If pets provide support, their owners would be expected to experience fewer or less extreme reactions to the stressful event. Conversely, the support model predicts that advantages to health and well-being should be less likely to be detected in studies of subject populations not specifically experiencing stressful circumstances, especially studies of a short duration, which are unlikely to pick up many periods of stress. If companionship from pets is important, however, Rook's (1990) theory would predict enhanced well-being even in pet owners who were not experiencing stressful events. To distinguish the consequences of different support processes and companionship processes, it is important to monitor the types of experiences and perceptions that owners have of their pets.

There are a number of hypotheses on how pets may function as providers of social support (McNicholas & Collis, 1995). Pets are perceived as always available, predictable in their responses, and nonjudgmental. They provide a sense of esteem in that pets are perceived as both caring about their owners, and needing them, regardless of the owner's status as perceived by self or others. Pets can also give tactile comfort and recreational distraction from worries. Pets are less subject to provider burnout. Thus, they may be a consistent source of support regardless of fluctuations in human support. No social skills are required to elicit attention from pets, whereas in human-human relationships, there is the issue of assessing how best to mobilize support. Because social competence in negotiating or regulating social support is less of an issue with pets, there may be a reduced likelihood of mismatches between required and received support or perceived shortfalls in received support. Pets may provide a refuge from the strains of human interactions, allowing a freedom from pretenses or barriers that may necessarily be erected between giver and recipient of support to mutually protect the relationship.

Thus, there is a compelling story to be told about how effective pets might be as sources of support. Unfortunately, the empirical evidence to support this story is lacking. To examine the hypothesis that pets convey advantages to human health and well-being via the provision of support, there needs to be a careful evaluation of how these components of support, separately or in combination, predict individual differences in health, well-being, or resilience in the face of adversity.

Social Support as an Explanation for Physiological Effects

The basic paradigm in this research is to measure blood pressure, heart rate, and similar variables to establish baseline levels and then to take similar measurements during the performance of a task known to produce stresslike changes in these physiological indexes. Such a procedure is taken as a laboratory model for responses to relatively minor stressors in everyday life. Factors that influence responses to stress in the laboratory might be expected to influence responses in real life—hence the ability to predict susceptibility to stress-related disease such as cardiovascular disease, arising from the cumulative effects of responses to everyday stressors (Steptoe, 1990). In the companion animal literature, the focus is on the role of an animal, usually a dog, in ameliorating cardiovascular responses to stress (Friedmann, 1995). An explicit link is often made with studies reporting that pet ownership is associated with advantages in cardiovascular health (Anderson et al., 1992; Friedmann et al., 1980). The paradigm is logical, however, only where it is possible to demonstrate the effects of a companion animal on the changes in physiological indexes between baseline and stress phases or, equivalently, a statistical interaction between condition (animal present or absent) and phase (baseline versus task). In some studies, statistical interactions are noticeable by their absence, and only main effects of condition are available for interpretation (e.g., Friedmann, Katcher, Thomas, Lynch, & Messent, 1983). This may be a consequence of baseline periods being too brief to provide stable estimates of true baseline levels of cardiovascular activity (Shapiro et al., 1996), or it may that the stress-reduction effect of the animal is either absent or too weak to be detected.

When the presence of a companion animal is shown to influence cardiovascular response to stress, what sort of processes might be operating? Is this an instance of social support in action? Are there alternative explanations? First, the animal might be acting as a social catalyst in smoothing the social encounter between the participants and experimenter, reducing the level of stress in the human-human interaction. This would be an indirect causal effect. Second, it has been repeatedly suggested that the mere presence of an animal could reduce stress responses as a direct effect (Friedmann, 1995). This possibility could be accommodated within the arousal theory of social facilitation (Allen, Blascovich, Tomaka, & Kelsey, 1991), but it is not particularly helpful to characterize such an effect as involving the provision of support.

Third, the key factor might be interaction with the animal. Stress-reducing effects of minimal interaction with a human friend in laboratory settings have been described as social support (Kamarck, Manuck, & Jennings, 1990), but there are a number of reasons why this does not seem to be the same type of process that is labeled social support in the health psychology and epidemiology literature. Social support is believed to be effective in a broader range of contexts than the prevention of cardiovascular disease. The time scale of effects in this experimental paradigm seems quite different from the classic interpretation of social support. The more powerful aspects of support, especially emotional and esteem support, are thought to depend on a supportive relationship based on a degree of mutual understanding, rather than just supportive communication in the current, stressful experience. At best, effects of positive communication from confederates previously unknown to participants (Sheffield & Carroll, 1996) need to be clearly distinguished from effects arising from expectations about the attitude of the others toward oneself based on a relationship established by a history of interaction. Success in unraveling these complex issues will require an analysis of cognitive representations of perceived support. The study by Allen et al. (1991) implies that the presence of friends might increase stress responses in the immediate context of a laboratory stress task because they are perceived as evaluative. This is not incompatible, however, with a view of supportive relationships that suggests that during a longer time, support from friends should be particularly effective in ameliorating the effects of stress. Allen et al. interpreted the role of dogs in short-term laboratory studies as nonevaluative friends, but it is not clear how they were perceived by the participants.

References

Ainsworth, M. D. S. (1989). Attachments beyond infancy. *American Psychologist, 44,* 709-716.

Allen, K. M., Blascovich, J., Tomaka, J. & Kelsey, R. M. (1991). Presence of human friends and pet dogs as moderators of autonomic responses to stress in women. *Journal of Personality and Social Psychology, 61,* 582-589.

Anderson, W. P., Reid, C. M., & Jennings, G. L. (1992). Pet ownership and risk factors for cardiovascular disease. *Medical Journal of Australia, 157,* 298-301.

Archer, J., & Winchester, G. (1993). Bereavement following death of a pet. *British Journal of Psychology, 85,* 259-271.

Bowlby, J. (1969). *Attachment.* Harmondsworth, UK: Penguin.

Bowlby, J. (1979). *The making and breaking of affectional bonds.* London: Tavistock.

Bretherton, I. (1985). Attachment theory: Retrospect and prospect. *Monographs for the Society for Research in Child Development, 50,* 3-35.

Bretherton, I. (1987). New perspectives on attachment relations: Security, communication and internal working models. In J. D. Osofsky (Ed.), *Handbook of infant development* (2nd ed., pp. 106-110). New York: John Wiley.

Cobb, S. (1976). Social support as a moderator of life stress. *Psychosomatic Medicine, 38,* 300-314.

Cohen, S., & Wills, T. A. (1985). Stress, social support, and the buffering hypothesis. *Psychological Bulletin, 98,* 310-357.

Crowell, J. A., & Treboux, D. (1995). A review of adult attachment measures: Implications for theory and research. *Social Development, 4,* 294-327.

Cutrona, C. E., & Russell, D. W. (1990). Type of social support and specific stress: Toward a theory of optimal matching. In B. R. Sarason, I. G. Sarason, & G. R. Pierce (Eds.), *Social support: An interactional view* (pp. 319-366). New York: John Wiley.

Fontana, A. F., Kerns, R. D., Rosenberg, R. L., & Colonese, K. L. (1989). Support, stress and recovery from coronary heart disease: A longitudinal causal model. *Health Psychology, 8,* 175-193.

Friedmann, E. (1995). The role of pets in enhancing human well-being: Physiological effects. In I. Robinson (Ed.), *The Waltham book of human-animal interaction: Benefits and responsibilities of pet ownership* (pp. 33-53). Oxford, UK: Pergamon.

Friedmann, E., Katcher, A. H., Lynch, J. J., & Thomas, S. A. (1980). Animal companions and one year survival of patients after discharge from a coronary care unit. *Public Health Reports, 95,* 307-312.

Friedmann, E., Katcher, A. H., Thomas, S. A., Lynch, J. J., & Messent, P. R. (1983). Social interaction and blood pressure: The influence of animal companions. *Journal of Nervous and Mental Disease, 171,* 461-465.

George, C. (1996). A representational perspective of child abuse and prevention: Internal working models of attachment and caregiving. *Child Abuse and Neglect, 20,* 411-424.

Glass, T. A., Matchar, D. B., Belyea, M., & Feussner, J. R. (1993). Impact of social support on outcome in first stroke. *Stroke, 24,* 64-70.

Harlow, H. F., & Harlow, M. R. (1965). The affectional systems. In A. M. Schrier, H. F. Harlow, & F. Stollnitz (Eds.), *Behavior of non-human primates* (Vol. 2, pp. 287-334). New York: Academic Press.

Hazan, C., & Shaver, P. R. (1987). Romantic love conceptualized as an attachment process. *Journal of Personality and Social Psychology, 52,* 511-524.

Herzog, H. A., & Burghardt, G. M. (1987). Are we ready for a theory of human-animal relations? *Anthrozoös, 1,* 145-146.

Hinde, R. A. (1966). *Animal behavior.* New York: McGraw-Hill.

Holcombe, R., Williams, R. C., & Richards, P. S. (1985). The elements of attachment: Relationship maintenance and intimacy. *Journal of the Delta Society, 2*(1), 28-34.

Johnson, T. P., Garrity, T. F., & Stallones, L. (1991). Psychometric evaluation of the Lexington Attachment to Pets Scale (LAPS). *Anthrozoös, 5,* 160-175.

Kamarck, T. W., Manuck, S. B., & Jennings, B. R. (1990). Social support reduces cardiovascular reactivity to psychological challenge: A laboratory model. *Psychosomatic Medicine, 52,* 42-58.

Klaus, M. H., & Kennell, J. H. (1976). *Maternal-infant bonding.* St. Louis, MO: C. V. Mosby.

Kulik, J. A., & Mahler, H. I. M. (1993). Emotional support as a moderator of adjustment and compliance after coronary artery bypass surgery: A longitudinal study. *Journal of Behavioral Medicine, 16,* 45-63.

Main, M., Caplan, N., & Cassidy, J. (1985). Security in infancy, childhood, and adulthood: A move to the level of representation. *Monographs for the Society for Research in Child Development, 50,* 66-104.

McNicholas, J., & Collis, G. M. (1995). The end of a relationship: Coping with pet loss. In I. Robinson (Ed.), *The Waltham book of human-animal interaction: Benefits and responsibilities of pet ownership* (pp. 127-143). Oxford, UK: Pergamon.

McNicholas, J., Collis, G. M., Morley, I. E., & Lane, D. R. (1993). Social communication through a companion animal: The dog as a social catalyst. In M. Nichelmann, H. K. Wierenga, & S. Braun (Eds.), *Proceedings of the International Congress on Applied Ethology* (pp. 368-370). Berlin, Germany: Humboldt University.

Messent, P. R. (1983). Social facilitation of contact with other people by pet dogs. In A. H. Katcher & A. M. Beck (Eds.), *New perspectives on our lives with companion animals* (pp. 45-67). Philadelphia: University of Philadelphia Press.

Mugford, R. A., & M'Comisky, J. G. (1975). Some recent work on the psychotherapeutic value of caged birds with old people. In R. S. Anderson (Ed.), *Pets, animals and society* (pp. 54-65). London: Bailliere Tindall.

Myers, B. J. (1984). Mother-infant bonding: The status of this critical period hypothesis. *Developmental Review, 4,* 240-274.

Poresky, R. H., Hendrix, C., Mosier, J. E., & Samuelson, M. L. (1987). The companion animal bonding scale. *Psychological Reports, 60,* 743-746.

Rajaram, S. S., Garrity, T. F., Stallones, L., & Marx, M. B. (1993). Bereavement: Loss of a pet and loss of a human. *Anthrozoös, 6,* 8-16.

Rook, K. S. (1990). Social relationships as a source of companionship. In B. R. Sarason, I. G. Sarason, & G. R. Pierce (Eds.), *Social support: An interactional view*. New York: John Wiley.

Sarason, B. R., Pierce, G. R., & Sarason, I. G. (1990). Social support: The sense of acceptance and the role of relationships. In B. R. Sarason, I. G. Sarason, & G. R. Pierce (Eds.), *Social support: An interactional view*. New York: John Wiley.

Serpell, J. (1987). In defense of ethology. *Anthrozoös, 1,* 152-153.

Serpell, J. (1991). Beneficial effects of pet ownership on some aspects of human health and behaviour. *Journal of the Royal Society of Medicine, 84,* 717-720.

Shapiro, D., Jamner, L. D., Lane, J. D., Light, K. C., Myrtek, M., Sawada, Y., & Steptoe, A. (1996). Blood pressure publication guidelines. *Psychophysiology, 33,* 1-12.

Sheffield, D., & Carroll, D. (1996). Task-induced cardiovascular activity and the presence of a supportive or undermining other. *Psychology and Health, 11,* 583-591.

Siegel, J. M. (1990). Stressful life events and use of physician services among the elderly: The moderating role of pet ownership. *Journal of Personality and Social Psychology, 58,* 1081-1086.

Sluckin, W., Herbert, M., & Sluckin, A. (1983). *Maternal bonding*. Oxford, UK: Blackwell.

Sperling, W. H., & Berman, M. B. (1994). *Attachment in adults: Clinical and developmental perspectives*. New York: Guilford.

Steptoe, A. (1990). The value of mental stress testing in the investigation of cardiovascular disorders. In L. R. Schmidt, P. Schwenkmezger, J. Weinman, & S. Maes (Eds.), *Theoretical and applied aspects of health psychology*. Chur, Switzerland: Harwood Academic.

Weiss, R. S. (1974). The provisions of social relationships. In Z. Rubin (Ed.), *Doing unto others* (pp. 17-26). Englewood Cliffs, NJ: Prentice Hall.

Weiss, R. S. (1982). Attachment in adult life. In C. M. Parkes & J. Stevenson-Hinde (Eds.), *The place of attachment in human behavior* (pp. 171-184). New York: Basic Books.

West, M. L., & Sheldon-Keller, A. E. (1994). *Patterns of relating: An adult attachment perspective*. New York: Guilford.

Wortman, C. B. (1984). Social support and the cancer patient: Conceptual and methodological issues. *Cancer, 53,* 2339-2360.

Wright, J. C., & Moore, D. (1982). Comments on animal companions and one year survival of patients after discharge. *Public Health Reports, 97,* 380-381.

Zwick, W. R., & Velicer, W. F. (1986). Comparison of five rules for determining the number of components to retain. *Psychological Bulletin, 99,* 432-442.

Loneliness, Stress, and Human-Animal Attachment Among Older Adults **7**

Carolyn P. Keil

Abstract

The purpose of this descriptive study was to explore the role of human-animal bonding in quality of life of older adults. More specifically, the relationships among pet attachment, loneliness, and stress were evaluated in animal owners ($N = 275$) from three community programs for older adults in the midwestern United States. Measures included the Human-Animal Relationship Questionnaire for attachment and two Revised Philadelphia Geriatric Center Morale Scale factors for loneliness and stress. Pearson correlations between attachment and loneliness ($r = .18, p = .002$) and between attachment and stress ($r = .30, p = .001$) indicated that as loneliness and stress increased, attachment increased. Visual interaction, dog ownership, stress, and the animal's appeal explained 31% of the variance of human-animal attachment, $F (4, 269) = 29.24, p = .001$. The correlation between loneliness and attachment was higher for participants without a human confidant. These findings suggested that animals could become supplementary attachment figures for older people.

AUTHOR'S NOTE: I thank Roma Lee Taunton, RN, Ph.D., Associate Professor of Nursing, University of Kansas, for her valuable assistance with this dissertation research. Correspondence regarding this chapter and Keil's Human-Animal Relationship Questionnaire (copyright 1990, available from the author) should be addressed to Carolyn P. Keil, R.N., Ph.D., 3211 Providence Drive, School of Nursing, University of Alaska, Anchorage, AK 99508.

Introduction

In the United States, the number of older adults is increasing, and they are experiencing a parallel increase in needs and concerns for quality of life. Researchers and theorists have defined quality of life as a single, multidimensional construct characterized by internal or subjective feelings of well-being (Murphy & Kupshik, 1992; Sauer & Warland, 1982). In the *activity theory* of aging, gerontologists have proposed that as people age, their psychological and social needs remain unchanged. Older people who stay active and find substitutes for work and replacements for lost friendships have been found most satisfied with life (Havighurst, 1968). Lemon, Bengston, and Peterson (1972) found that the quality of relationships was more important in life satisfaction than the quantity. Longino and Kart's (1982) research supported the positive relationship between life satisfaction and informal activity with friends and family. One criticism of activity theory, however, has been that not all older adults have options for remaining active and reconstructing their lives by substitution (Kart, 1985). Companion animals could provide an accessible and acceptable option for continued activity in interpersonal relationships.

Two quality of life components, loneliness and stress, were selected for this study of the role of attachment to animals among older adults. Attachment has been related to decreased loneliness (Lynch, 1977), decreased stress and tension, and increased quality of life (Murphy & Kupshik, 1992; Strain & Chappell, 1982). In a study by Matthews (1986), older participants reported that the richness and interdependence of long-term friendship were difficult to replace because of their multiple losses, sensory deficits, mental changes, and mobility problems. Weiss (1984) discussed the importance of attachment and the need for supplementary relationships to prevent and to relieve the pain and stress of loneliness.

Researchers have found benefits from relationships with animals. Animals have reduced stress (Katcher, 1984), increased relaxation effects (Baun, Bergstrom, Langston, & Thoma, 1984; Wilson, 1991), and improved morale and decreased loneliness (Goldmeier, 1986; Lago, Delaney, Miller, & Grill, 1989; Robb, 1983). Siegel (1990) found that for older people who did not own animals, stressful life events resulted in more physician contacts, whereas stressed animal owners did not increase physician contacts. Ory and Goldberg (1983) found that attached pet owners and nonowners were happier than unattached pet owners. In the research of Garrity, Stallones, Marx, and Johnson (1989), older pet owners with few human confidants, who were attached to their pets, reported less depression and symptoms of illness than those who were unattached to their animals. Comparison of animal owners with nonowners has been characteristic of most research found in the literature, and attachment to animals recently has been included as a variable.

In 1987, the (U.S.) National Institutes of Health held a Technology Assessment Workshop to explore the health benefits of human-animal relationships. Their findings (1988) suggested that attachment to animals might be an important variable for study, particularly among those who have experienced reduced social ties with other humans, such as older adults. Human-animal attachment and human confidant status were included as variables in this study of loneliness and stress among older animal owners.

Purpose

The purpose of this research was to describe the relationships of the quality of life concepts of loneliness and stress to human-animal attachment among older people who owned animals. Interest in the potential of animals to become supplementary attachment figures and to provide older people a means of remaining active in interpersonal relationships was derived from attachment theory and the activity theory of aging.

Antecedents to attachment, for bonding between human mother and child (Bowlby, 1991; Klaus & Kennell, 1982), included sensory interaction using any of the five senses and appeal of appearance. The visual sensory interaction of gazing with one's animal and appearance appeal, along with type of animal, were examined in this exploration of attachment between humans and animals.

Definition of Terms

Loneliness was defined as an unpleasant and subjective feeling of dissatisfaction when social relationships are perceived as inadequate (Murphy & Kupshik, 1992; Peplau & Perlman, 1982). The study included two measures of loneliness: the "lonely dissatisfaction" factor of Lawton's (1972, 1975) Revised Geriatric Center Morale Scale and "human confidant status," indicated by the item, "I have at least one person that I can share my innermost feelings with."

Stress was defined as agitation or tension resulting from an emotional reaction (Lawton, 1972; Murphy & Kupshik, 1992). Stress was measured by the "agitation" factor of Lawton's (1972, 1975) Revised Geriatric Center Morale Scale.

The definitions of the antecedents to attachment were based on the work of Klaus and Kennell (1982). *Visual sensory interaction,* defined for the study as gazing with one's animal, was measured by one item, "My animal looks deep into my eyes." *Appeal of the animal's appearance* was defined as the owner's perception of an animal's physical attributes as appealing. Appeal was measured by one item, "I like the way my animal looks."

Human-animal attachment was defined as a hierarchical relationship between a human and an animal, which could be any living thing other than a plant or another human. The highest level of attachment included attitudes of friendship and reciprocity; human-animal attachment was measured by Keil's Human-Animal Relationship Questionnaire (Keil, 1990).

Research Questions

This research was guided by five questions: What are the relationships among (1) loneliness, (2) stress, (3) the visual sensory interaction of gazing with one's animal, (4) appeal of the animal's appearance, and (5) type of animal to human-animal attachment in older pet owners?

Method

Participants

The sample included only animal owners, from three community-based programs for older adults. To participate in these programs, people had to be at least 60 years or older or be a spouse of someone 60 or older. The largest group of participants ($n = 127$) was selected from a federally funded congregate meal program. The smallest group ($n = 29$) included the homebound meal recipients of the same program. The remaining participants were members of a program for active older adults ($n = 119$) sponsored by a local university.

The percentage of program users who owned animals (the inclusion criteria for the study) was determined for each group. Of the meal site attenders, 23% owned animals. Only 12% of the homebound had animals, and 29% of the university-sponsored active group owned animals. Agreement to participate in the study was high: 96% for the meal recipients and 81% for those who received mailed questionnaires. The three groups increased sample heterogeneity and provided sufficient size ($N = 275$) for moderate power of .80 to detect a small effect size of .30 (Cohen, 1977).

Settings

The study, conducted in a six-county region of a midwestern state, included both rural (population of 25,000 or less) and urban participants. Data were collected at multiple meal sites (16), homes of the homebound, and through mailed questionnaires to the active older adults.

Measurement of Variables

Each of the three summated scales (as measures of loneliness, stress, and attachment) included six items and had previously been evaluated for reliability and validity. Lawton's (1972, 1975) measures of loneliness and stress were selected over other instruments because they were brief, simple (dichotomously scored), and appropriate for self-administration and had been developed for use with an older sample (Sauer & Warland, 1982). In this study, the alpha reliabilities were .67 for the loneliness scale, .74 for stress, and .65 for attachment. Confidence in the attachment measure was increased by the Spearman-Brown split-half reliability of .71 and retest results ($r = .77, p < .001$). Prior psychometric evaluation of this instrument indicated support for face, content, and contrasted groups construct validity and a prior Cronbach's alpha reliability of .83.

Older participants were assumed to need protection from fatigue, so limitations were placed on questionnaire length and number of scoring options. All other variables were measured with one item each, dichotomously scored when possible. Variables included an additional loneliness item of human confidant status; animal variables of gazing, appeal, and type; the demographic and confounding variables of perceived health, gender, marital status, income, age, availability of transportation, and recent loss or change. Rural or urban residence was determined by meal site or residence zip code.

Procedure

A pilot study was conducted at three meal sites. On the basis of pilot responses, the instrument was further simplified for these older adults. Each animal item was positively worded, and the scoring options were reduced from four to two. Data collection proceeded at the remaining meal sites, the homes of homebound participants, and through mailed questionnaires to the active older adults. In all settings, the survey was self-administered. Six-week retest reliability of the attachment scale was determined by randomly selecting 50 participants from all three groups. The study conformed to approved procedures for protection of human participants. Data analysis included pilot study results. An alpha level of .05 was used for all statistical tests.

Results

Demographic characteristics of participants indicated that almost one fourth resided in a rural area (24%). Health was rated as good or excellent by almost two thirds (65%) of these older adults. A large majority was female (69%). More than half were currently married (53%), and only 4% had never been married. A 1989 income of less than $15,000 (U.S.) was reported by 44% of the sample. Ages of participants ranged from 52 to 91 years, with a mean age of 71. Two thirds (67%) were younger than 75, including 10 participants who were less than 60. Using chi-square goodness-of-fit tests, these participants were determined to be representative of the U.S. older adult population for study characteristics (Ebersole & Hess, 1990; National Center for Health Statistics, 1987; Schick, 1986). Lack of transportation was reported by 12 (4%) participants, and 168 (61%) reported important changes or losses within the last year.

If participants had more than one animal, they were asked about the animal for which they had the *most* feelings. Of the sample, 60% based their response on their dogs, and 36% responded about their cats. The other 4% responded about birds (5), fish (4), horses (1), and cow (1).

TABLE 7.1   **Pearson Correlation of Variables With Human-Animal Attachment**

Variable	n	r With Higher Attachment	p
Gazing	274	.41	< .001
Stress	270	.30	< .001
Income	245	−.23	< .001
Appeal	274	.20	< .001
Lonely	269	.18	.002
Marital	274	−.16	.003
Transportation	274	−.13	.015
Age	270	.11	.034
Health	274	−.11	.039
Confidant	273	−.09	.062

NOTE: Negative *r* indicates less of the variable is correlated with higher attachment (i.e., low income, never married, no transportation, poorer health, no confidant).
Positive *r* indicates more of the variable is correlated with higher attachment.

To determine the relationship of attachment to the variables (a) loneliness, (b) stress, (c) the visual sensory interaction of gazing with one's animal, and (d) appeal of the animal's appearance, Pearson product moment correlation coefficients were calculated (Table 7.1). Results indicated that attachment to animals was higher when participants lacked a human confidant and were lonely, were stressed, gazed with their animals, and thought their animals looked appealing. Of the loneliness, stress, gazing, and appeal variables, only human confidant status was not significantly related to attachment.

Also reported in Table 7.1 are the Pearson correlations for demographic variables with attachment. Marital status was collapsed into never married/ever married categories, based on similarities of mean attachment scores. Results indicated that those participants who were older, reported lower incomes, lack of transportation, and poor health; and had never been married were significantly more likely to be attached to their animals. Gender and recent change were not significantly related to attachment. The correlation between lonely dissatisfaction and attachment (Table 7.2) increased from .18 to .30 for the 26 participants who lacked a human confidant, although the difference between the group with and the group with-

TABLE 7.2   Pearson Correlation Between Attachment and
Loneliness by Confidant Support

Support	Attachment With Loneliness		
	n	r	p
Human confidant			
With	242	.18	.003
Without	26	.30	.069

TABLE 7.3   Mean Attachment Scores by Type of Animal ($N = 269$)

Species	n	M
Dog	160	3.98
Bird	5	3.20
Cat	98	3.01
Horse/cow	2	1.50
Fish	4	1.25

NOTE: Possible range of attachment scores = 0 to 6, the overall $M = 3.54$; $SD = 1.71$.

out a human confidant was not significant ($Z = -0.595$; critical $Z = 1.96$; $p > .05$).

To answer to the fifth research question regarding the type of animal the participant responded about, analysis of variance and Duncan's post hoc group comparisons were calculated, $F (4, 268) = 8.37$, $p = < .001$. Dog owners had the highest attachment scores (Table 7.3), which were significantly different only from the attachment means for horse/cow and fish owners, who scored the lowest. Bird, then cat owners, had middle attachment scores. Type of animal was dummy coded into "dog and other" and "cat plus bird and others" for entry into a regression equation.

Variables of interest that had a significant relationship with attachment, had a meaningful effect size of .20 or above (explaining at least 4% of the variance), and were without problematic intercorrelations with other variables were selected for regression on attachment. Human confidant status

TABLE 7.4   Summary of Hierarchical Regression Analysis for Variables on Human-Animal Attachment ($N = 275$)

Variables	$R^2\Delta$	F	b	Beta	SE
Gazing	.17	55.83*	1.30	.34	.053
Dog owner	.07	42.98*	.85	.24	.052
Stress	.04	34.95*	.19	.20	.053
Appeal	.02	29.24*	1.47	.15	.052

NOTE: R^2 for Step 4 = .31.
*$p < .01$.

was not significantly related to attachment. The correlation between the loneliness scale and attachment was significant, but the effect size ($r = .18$) was not considered meaningful. The intercorrelation between loneliness and stress ($r = .57$) was higher than the correlation of either variable with attachment and suggested a problem with multicollinearity. Therefore, neither loneliness variable was included in the regression equation.

A stepwise regression procedure was used to assess the impact of five variables (i.e., gazing, appeal, stress, and 2 dummy-coded type of animal variables) on level of human-animal attachment. With the exception of one dummy-coded type of animal variable, each variable entered the regression equation with a significant F (Table 7.4). The final $F (4, 269)$ of 29.24 was significant at less than .001. The R square change indicated that gazing with the animal explained 17% of the regressed variance of human-animal attachment, with dog ownership, stress, and appeal of the animal's appearance explaining an additional 13%. Together, these four variables explained 31% of the variance of human-animal attachment.

Conclusions and Implications

The visual sensory interaction of gazing with one's animal was important in the variance of attachment. For many, hearing and touch compensate for visual impairments and could affect the type of animal most appropriate for attachment relationships. Any of the five senses could be an antecedent to human-animal attachment (Klaus & Kennell, 1982) and, along with type of animal, should be explored in future research. Dogs were more involved in these attachment relationships, possibly because with dogs the perception of reciprocal friendships was easily developed or because dogs were the best at mutual gazing. Interaction with birds, whose owners had the second highest mean attachment scores in this study, showed potential that should be explored.

Participants in this study were slightly more likely to be attached if they liked the way their animals looked. This suggested that older adults should participate in the selection of their own animals.

Several participants wrote extra comments on their questionnaires, sent pictures of their animals, or called the researcher. These actions and the high participation rate (96% for meal recipients and 81% for those who received mailed questionnaires) suggested that these older people wanted to talk about their animals. Older people might be more willing to participate in other research if animal topics were included.

Results were affected by the use of one-item measures with dichotomous scoring, the self-administered paper-and-pencil survey format, the convenience sample, and the small number of participants for some categories. Only 26 participants reported lack of a human confidant, 11 responded about animals other than dogs or cats, and 12 had never married, which provided little confidence in these results. The inclusion of 10 participants under the age of 60 increased the potential for variance between subsamples. The low correlation between loneliness and attachment ($r = .18$) and between stress and attachment ($r = .30$) could have been due to the relatively low alpha reliabilities of the instruments. The findings did support that these variables and the methodological issues should be addressed in future research.

In a 7-year longitudinal study of pet ownership, Lago et al. (1989) reported that as health and morale decreased, affection for animals increased. In research in which owners were compared with nonowners (Goldmeier, 1986; Robb, 1983), ownership of animals was significantly related to improved quality of life, but attachment was not a variable in these studies. The research reported in this study explored attachment among animal owners and demonstrated that as quality of life deteriorated, attachment to animals increased. The study was limited by the absence of a nonowner control group. To describe loneliness, stress, and other quality of life variables as outcomes of attachment, future researchers should include nonowners.

These results contributed to the understanding of human-animal attachment and relationship of attachment to the quality of life variables of loneliness and stress. Study participants who gazed with their animals; owned dogs; thought their animals looked appealing; were lonely and stressed; were older; had never been married; and reported poor health, low income, and lack of transportation were more likely to be highly attached to their animals. The higher correlation between loneliness and attachment for those who lacked human confidants indicated that animals might have been an important resource for that group. These findings suggested that animals became supplementary attachment figures for the older adults who had the least resources to satisfy their needs. Attachment to animals as a resource to help disadvantaged older people remain active in reciprocal relationships and maintain quality of life has shown potential as an innovative strategy that warrants additional exploration.

References

Baun, M. M., Bergstrom, N., Langston, N. F., & Thoma, L. (1984). Physiological effects of human-companion animal bonding. *Nursing Research, 33,* 126-129.

Bowlby, J. (1991). Postscript. In C. M. Parkes, J. Stevenson-Hinde, & P. Marris (Eds.), *Attachment across the life cycle* (pp. 293-299). London: Tavistock/Routledge.

Cohen, J. (1977). *Statistical power analysis for the behavioral sciences.* New York: Academic Press.

Ebersole, P., & Hess, P. (1990). *Toward healthy aging.* St. Louis, MO: C. V. Mosby.

Garrity, T. F., Stallones, L., Marx, M. B., & Johnson, T. P. (1989). Pet ownership and attachment as supportive factors in the health of the elderly. *Anthrozoös, 3,* 35-44.

Goldmeier, J. (1986). Pets or people: Another research note. *Gerontologist, 26*(2), 203-206.

Havighurst, R. (1968). Personality and patterns of aging. *Gerontologist, 8,* 20-23.

Kart, C. S. (1985). *The realities of aging.* Boston: Allyn & Bacon.

Katcher, A. H. (1984). Emotional and cognitive responses to interaction with companion animals. *Journal of the Delta Society, 1,* 34-36.

Keil, C. I. P. (1990). *Conceptual framework of human-animal relationships: An empirical examination.* Lawrence: University of Kansas. (UMI order 3 PUZ9119085)

Klaus, M. H., & Kennell, J. H. (1982). *Parent-infant bonding.* St. Louis, MO: C. V. Mosby.

Lago, D., Delaney, M., Miller, M., & Grill, C. (1989). Companion animals, attitudes toward pets, and health outcomes among the elderly: A long-term follow-up. *Anthrozoös, 3,* 25-34.

Lawton, M. P. (1972). The dimensions of morale. In D. P. Kent, R. Kastenbaum, & S. Sherwood (Eds.), *Research planning and action for the elderly: The power and potential of social science* (pp. 144-165). New York: Behavioral Publications.

Lawton, M. P. (1975). The Philadelphia Geriatric Center Morale Scale: A revision. *Journal of Gerontology, 30,* 85-89.

Lemon, B. W., Bengston, V. L., & Peterson, J. A. (1972). An exploration of the activity theory of aging: Activity types and life satisfaction among in-movers to a retirement community. *Journal of Gerontology, 27,* 511-523.

Longino, C. F., & Kart, C. S. (1982). Explicating activity theory: A formal replication. *Journal of Gerontology, 37*(6), 713-722.

Lynch, J. J. (1977). *The broken heart: The medical consequences of loneliness.* New York: Basic Books.

Matthews, S. H. (1986). Friendships in old age: Biography and circumstances. In V. W. Marshall (Ed.), *Later life: The social psychology of aging* (pp. 233-269). Beverly Hills, CA: Sage.

Murphy, P. M., & Kupshik, G. A. (1992). *Loneliness, stress and well-being: A helper's guide.* London: Tavistock/Routledge.

National Center for Health Statistics. (1987). *Health statistics on older persons, United States, 1986: Vital and health statistics.* (Series 3, No. 25; DHHS Publication No. PHS 87-1409). Washington, DC: Government Printing Office.

National Institutes of Health. (1988). *National Institutes of Health Technology Assessment workshop: Health benefits of pets* (DHHS Publication No. 88-216-107). Washington, DC: Government Printing Office.

Ory, M. G., & Goldberg, E. L. (1983). Pet possession and life satisfaction in elderly women. In A. H. Katcher & A. M. Beck (Eds.), *New perspectives on our lives with companion animals* (pp. 303-317). Philadelphia: University of Pennsylvania Press.

Peplau, L. A., & Perlman, D. (Eds.). (1982). *Loneliness: A sourcebook of current theory, research and therapy.* New York: John Wiley.

Robb, S. S. (1983). Health status correlates of pet-human association in a health-impaired population. In A. H. Katcher & A. M. Beck (Eds.), *New perspectives on our lives with companion animals* (pp. 318-327). Philadelphia: University of Pennsylvania Press.

Sauer, W. J., & Warland, R. (1982). Morale and life satisfaction. In D. J. Mangen & W. A. Peterson (Eds.), *Research instruments in social gerontology: Clinical and Social Psychology,* Vol. 1 (pp. 195-240). Minneapolis: University of Minnesota Press.

Schick, F. (Ed.). (1986). *Statistical handbook on aging Americans.* Phoenix, AZ: Onyx.

Siegel, J. M. (1990). Stressful life events and use of physician services among the elderly: The moderating role of pet ownership. *Journal of Personality and Social Psychology, 13,* 1081-1086.

Strain, L. A., & Chappell, N. L. (1982). Confidants: Do they make a difference in quality of life? *Research on Aging, 4,* 479-502.

Weiss, R. S. (1984). Loneliness. In L. A. Peplau & S. E. Goldston (Eds.), *Preventing the harmful consequences of severe and persistent loneliness* (pp. 3-12). Rockville, MD: U.S. Department of Health and Human Services, National Institute of Mental Health.

Wilson, C. C. (1991). The pet as an anxiolytic intervention. *Journal of Nervous and Mental Disease, 179,* 482-489.

The Relationship Between Attachment to Companion Animals and Self-Esteem

8

A Developmental Perspective

Sandra Lookabaugh Triebenbacher

Abstract

Developmental differences in the relationship between children's attachment to companion animals and their self-esteem were investigated. Participation in the study was open to any child returning a completed permission form, regardless of current pet ownership. The sample included 436 children (232 boys and 204 girls) in grades 4 through 12; 88% were currently pet owners, and 12% were not pet owners. Only the responses from current pet owners ($N = 385$) were included in data analysis. Attachment to companion animals was measured using the Companion Animal Bonding Scale developed by Poresky, Hendrix, Mosier, and Samuelson (1987). Global self-esteem was measured using the New York Self-Esteem Scale/Rosenberg Self-Esteem Scale developed by Rosenberg (1979). The results indicated developmental differences in children's attachment to their companion animals and their self-esteem ratings. The results are discussed as direct and indirect relationships between attachment to companion animals and self-esteem ratings.

The contributions companion animals make to the emotional well-being of humans are well documented and include (a) providing noncontingent unconditional love and opportunities for love and affection; (b) functioning as a friend, confidant, playmate, and companion; (c) serving as a living transitional object; and (d) assisting in the achievement of trust, autonomy, responsibility, competence, and empathy toward others (Beck & Katcher, 1983; Kidd & Kidd, 1985; Levinson, 1972; Robin & ten Bensel, 1985; Triebenbacher, 1994). An individual's self-esteem is another dimension of emotional well-being that could be enhanced by the presence of and attachment to a companion animal. To explore the potential relationship between attachment to companion animals and self-esteem, a blending of theoretical frameworks is necessary.

Understanding the attachment relationship between humans and animals draws on literature describing human-to-human attachment (Ainsworth, 1969; Bowlby, 1969) and animal-to-animal attachment (Harlow & Zimmerman, 1959). Attachment is described as an "affectional tie that one person (or animal) forms to another specific individual," and although attachment behaviors may vary according to situational factors, attachments endure across space and time (Ainsworth, 1969, p. 971). The enduring emotional bond and the reciprocal nature of the attachment relationship are central components defining attachment theory.

An important function of the human attachment figures is to serve as a secure base from which children can explore the world (Ainsworth, 1982). Through extrapolation from human attachment theory, the idea that companion animals may also serve as a secure base for children appears plausible. The unconditional love and acceptance and sense of security conveyed in the human-animal attachment relationship may validate a child's sense of self-worth and facilitate a positive attitude toward the self. Given the unconditional love and acceptance proposed in the human-animal attachment relationship, can one make the theoretical proposition that children who feel unconditionally loved and accepted by their companion animal also feel a sense of love and acceptance toward themselves?

The literature on self-esteem yielded little consensus about the conceptualization, operational definition, and measurement of self-esteem (Demo, 1985). Self-esteem has been viewed both as a differentiated, fluctuating self-attitude and as a global characteristic (Harter, 1983). Harter views self-esteem as a fluctuating self-attitude reflecting changing roles, expectations, performances, responses from others, and other situational characteristics. This view of self-esteem is considered specific self-esteem. Rosenberg (1979) and Coopersmith (1967) are proponents of the global nature of self-esteem, in which self-esteem is viewed as a personality trait characterized by considerable stability from one situation to the next and is defined as an overall positive or negative attitude toward the self. Global self-esteem "appears to be heavily affective in nature and tends to be associated with overall psychological well-being" (Rosenberg, Schooler, Schoenbach, & Rosenberg, 1995, p. 153). The affective nature of the global self-esteem perspective appears be relevant and useful in understanding the relationship between children's attachment to companion animals and their overall attitude toward the self.

The concepts defining attachment and self-esteem theory appear to be compatible and may offer new insight into the complexity of human-animal relations. The purpose of the present study was to propose a conceptual framework that combines the theoretical and empirical elements of human-animal attachment and self-esteem and examine the relationship between attachment to companion animals (pets) and self-esteem among children at different developmental levels. Secondary research questions examine the role of gender and pet type in the relationship between attachment to companion animals and self-esteem.

Method

Participants

In a public school district in a metropolitan area, 436 children (232 boys and 204 girls) enrolled in grades 4 through 12 volunteered for participation. The total sample included 364 Caucasians (84%) and 72 members of other racial and other ethnic groups (16%), consisting of African Americans, Latinos, Asian Americans, and biracial individuals. Of the total sample, 86% (n = 385) were pet owners, and 12% (n = 51) were not pet owners. The sample demographics are presented in Table 8.1.

Measures and Coding

All participants completed a demographic questionnaire developed for this study to obtain information about age, gender, grade, ethnic group, pet ownership, type of pet(s), and length of pet ownership. The Companion

TABLE 8.1   Demographics of Child Participants

Characteristic	Elementary (33%) Grades 4-6 n = 146	Middle (34%) Grades 7-9 n = 148	High (33%) Grades 10-12 n = 142
Mean age	11 yrs. (.92)	14 yrs. (.65)	16 yrs. (1.08)
Age range	11-13 yrs.	13-15 yrs.	15-18 yrs.
Gender			
Boys	78	76	78
Girls	68	72	64
Ethnic group			
Caucasian	125	125	114
Other	21	23	28
Pet ownership			
Yes	130	128	127
No	16	20	15
Pet type			
Dog	82	75	69
Cat	29	28	45
Other[a]	19	25	13
Mean length of ownership	3 yrs. (3.01)	3 yrs. (2.73)	4.5 yrs. (3.35)

NOTES: $N = 436$ (completing questionnaires); $N = 385$ (responses used in data analysis); Standard deviation in parentheses.
a. Bird, reptile, rodent, or horse.

Animal Bonding Scale (CABS; Poresky, Hendrix, Mosier, & Samuelson, 1987) and the New York Self-Esteem Scale/Rosenberg Self-Esteem Scale (RSE; Rosenberg, 1979) were also completed.

Dependent Variables

Attachment to companion animals was measured using the CABS. This eight-item questionnaire uses a five-point Likert format (1 = *never;* 2 = *rarely;* 3 = *often;* 4 = *generally;* 5 = *always*) to assess self-reported behavior indicative of a bond between a person and an animal. The CABS was selected as the measurement for attachment to companion animals because the items ask behavioral questions such as "How often does your companion animal sleep in your room?" that are considered to be more objective than a more general and subjective question such as "How attached are you to your companion animal?" The reported internal reliability of the scale was a Cronbach alpha of .77 (Poresky et al., 1987).

Self-esteem was measured using the New York Self-Esteem Scale/Rosenberg Self-Esteem Scale (RSE). The RSE is a 10-item Guttman Scale (1 = *strongly disagree;* 2 = *disagree;* 3 = *agree;* 4 = *strongly agree*) to measure global self-esteem. This measure was selected as a measure of general self-worth, beyond specific attributes in specific contexts. The RSE is reported to have a reliability coefficient of .92 (Rosenberg, 1979).

Independent Variables

The variable of *types of pet* was classified into two categories: "cat/dog" and "other." Preliminary analyses revealed no significant differences between cat and dog owners on the CABS and RSE; therefore, these two pet types were combined. The small percentage of pets other than cats and dogs (15%) were combined for the second category of "other." The variable of *gender* of the child participant was coded as a dichotomous variable.

Procedures

Permission to conduct research was obtained from the assessment and evaluation division, principals, teachers, parents, and children in a public school system located in a metropolitan area on the East Coast. Schools were randomly selected within the school district, and participation in the study was open to all children, regardless of pet ownership, in the participating schools. Only those children agreeing to participate and receiving parental permission were included in the study.

Completion of all questionnaires occurred in the classroom, using group administration techniques. For elementary participants, each item on the three measures was read to the students, and they responded independently to each item. Middle and high school participants independently read and responded to each item on the three measures. Responses to CABS items by current pet owners reflected attachment to their most significant pet, whereas responses by non-pet-owning participants were hypothetical (i.e., if they were a pet owner). All participant responses were anonymous in an attempt to decrease the likelihood of socially desirable responses and increase the chances of honest replies. Only those responses from current pet owners ($N = 385$) were used in this data analysis.

Data Analysis

Path analysis using LISREL submodel 2 was used for data analysis. This statistical procedure is appropriate when examining causal relationships. Path analysis measures both direct (causal relationships between two variables) and indirect (compound causal relationships with an intervening variable) effects, while examining a series of dependent relationships simultaneously. A recursive model and linear relationships are assumed. No chi-square goodness-of-fit estimates are provided because the path model is perfectly identified (i.e., all paths are released). Overall measures of fit are not appropriate because the focus of this study was not to test theory but rather to build and develop theoretical propositions related to children's attachment to companion animals and their self-esteem (Bollen, 1989).

Correlation matrices, means, and standard deviations for variables in the self-esteem path analysis models are illustrated in Table 8.2. Regression statistics for variables in the path analysis models are included in Figures 8.1 through 8.4.

Results

Path analysis was performed to examine (a) direct effects of gender and type of pet on attachment to companion animal and self-esteem rating and (b) indirect effects of gender and type of pet on self-esteem via attachment to companion animal. The path analysis diagrams depict overall statistical results (Figure 8.1: Full Model), including information from all participants considered simultaneously, as well as separate path analysis diagrams for the elementary, middle, and high school populations (Figures 8.2 through 8.4: Elementary, Middle, and High School Models), allowing for interpretation of developmental differences. Path coefficients, numerical estimates of the causal relationship, are noted on each path in the four models.

TABLE 8.2 Correlation Matrices, Means, and Standard Deviations of Variables in Self-Esteem Path Analysis

Variable	Mean (SD)	1	2	3	4
1. RSE	31.70 (5.42)[a]	—	.1545**	.0954	−.1303**
	32.02 (4.40)[b]	—	.1348	.1303	.2990**
	31.65 (5.33)[c]	—	−.0161	.0127	−.1189
	31.43 (6.39)[d]	—	.3417**	.1815*	.2316**
2. CABS	28.82 (6.05)[d]	—	—	.2527*	.1264**
	27.34 (6.23)[d]	—	—	.3938**	.2990**
	27.35 (5.64)[d]	—	—	.2038**	−.0300
	29.82 (6.03)[d]	—	—	.1479	.0666
3. Pet type		—	—	—	−.0541
		—	—	—	−.0466
		—	—	—	−.0498
		—	—	—	−.0460
4. Sex		—	—	—	—

NOTE: RSE = Rosenberg Self-Esteem Scale; CABS = Companion Animal Bonding Scale.
a. Total group (**N** = 385).
b. Elementary school (*n* = 130).
c. Middle school (*n* = 128).
d. High school (*n* = 127).
*p < .05; **p < .01.

The path analysis for the full model (Figure 8.1) revealed that children with a cat or dog were significantly more attached to their companion animal than were children with other types of companion animals such as a bird, reptile, rodent, or horse (*p* < .01) and that girls were significantly more attached to their companion animals than were boys (*p* < .01). The path analysis for the full model revealed no direct effect (i.e., no causal relationship) between pet ownership and self-esteem. Type of pet (cat or dog) and gender (girl) were indirectly related to self-esteem via attachment as the intervening variable with the path coefficient = .161.

As revealed in the full model, type of pet was directly related to attachment at the elementary (path coefficient = .409), middle (path coefficient = .203), and high (path coefficient = .151) school levels. At each developmental level, children with a cat or dog were more attached to their

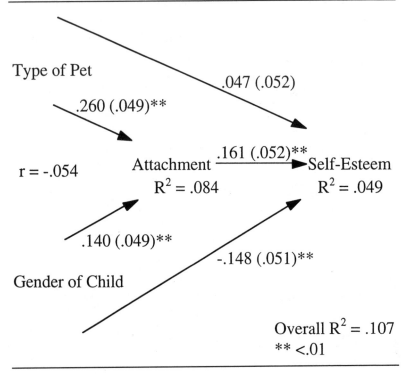

Figure 8.1. Full Model
NOTE: Relationships between pet type, gender of child, attachment to pet, and self-esteem rating for the total group. Standardized regression coefficients (path coefficients) followed by the standard errors in parentheses are noted on each path in the model.

companion animal than were children with a bird, reptile, rodent, or horse ($p < .01$). At the high school level, type of pet (cat or dog) was indirectly related to self-esteem via attachment (path coefficient = .341). The separate path analysis models (Figures 8.2 through 8.4) revealed gender differences at the elementary and high school levels. Elementary school girls were significantly more attached to their companion animals than were boys ($p < .01$), and boys at the high school level reported significantly higher self-esteem than did high school girls ($p < .01$).

The proportion of explained variance (R^2) for all four models (full, elementary, middle, and high school models) was .107, .262, .056, to .114, respectively. The greatest amount of explained variance was in the elemen-

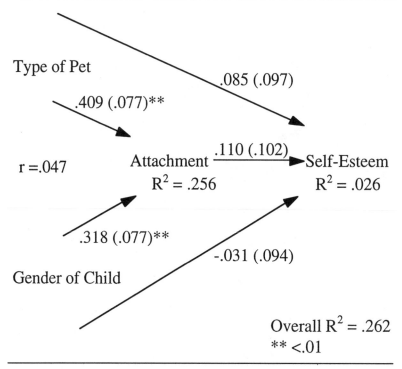

Figure 8.2. Elementary School Model
NOTE: Relationships between pet type, gender of child, attachment to pet, and self-esteem rating for the elementary school population. Standardized regression coefficients (path coefficients) followed by the standard errors in parentheses are noted on each path in the model.

tary school model, whereas the least amount was explained in the middle school model.

Discussion

Results of this study reveal that children's attachment to a companion animal is positively related to their sense of self-esteem. Relationships between gender of child, type of pet, attachment to companion animals, and self-esteem rating are discussed, along with suggestions for future research.

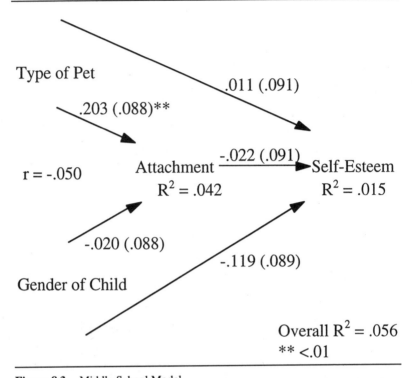

Figure 8.3. Middle School Model
NOTE: Relationships between pet type, gender of child, attachment to pet, and self-esteem rating for the middle school population. Standardized regression coefficients (path coefficients) followed by the standard errors in parentheses are noted on each path in the model.

At all developmental levels, children with interactive pets such as cats and dogs were more attached to their companion animals than were children with other types of pets (i.e., a direct relationship between pet type and attachment). Given the reciprocal influences in attachment relationships, humans may be more likely to form an emotional bond to animals that are able to respond to them in outwardly loving and affectionate ways. Melson (1988) describes dogs and cats as more interactive companion animals and hamsters, fish, and turtles as less interactive. The responsiveness and proximity-seeking behaviors of cats and dogs, as shown through purring, tail wagging, barking, and initiation to be petted, may be classified by humans as attachment behaviors, whereas other types of pets may elicit different responses in their human caregivers. An animal's unconditional

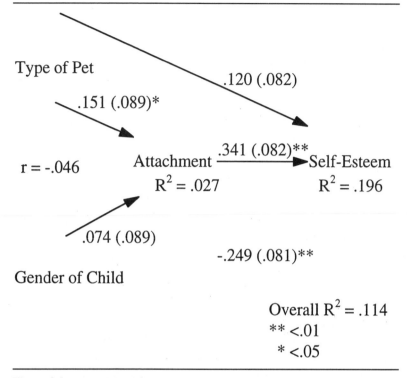

Figure 8.4. High School Model
NOTE: Relationships between pet type, gender of child, attachment to pet, and self-esteem rating for the high school population. Standardized regression coefficients (path coefficients) followed by the standard errors in parentheses are noted on each path in the model.

love, companionship, and commitment to its human caregiver may be perceived and interpreted in a variety ways. Pet owners of exotic pets, rodents, and horses accounted for such a small percentage ($n = 57$) of the sample that interpretation of this research finding should be viewed in the context of human relationships with cats and dogs.

Consistent with existing literature regarding gender differences in attachment to companion animals (Holcomb, Williams, & Richards, 1985; Melson & Fogle, 1989; Stevens, 1990), this study revealed few gender differences. Stevens states that discrepancies of gender differences in pet attachment could be attributed to methodological design. In this study, elementary school girls were significantly more attached to their companion animals than were boys, which could be partially explained by gender role socialization early in life. One can postulate that affection and nurturance of companion animals are inherent aspects of the human-animal relationship across development regardless of gender, although further exploration of gender similarities and differences is warranted.

Boys at the high school level reported significantly higher self-esteem ratings than did girls at the high school level, thus a direct relationship between gender and self-esteem ratings. This finding is consistent with the literature surrounding self-esteem in adolescence (Abramowitz, Peterson, & Schulenberg, 1984; Block & Robins, 1993). In general, gender differences in self-esteem ratings have been attributed to a myriad of factors, including gender role socialization as well as unique, individual variations.

Although there was no direct relationship between pet type and self-esteem ratings at any developmental level, an indirect relationship emerged at the high school level. Attachment to a cat or dog was indirectly related to self-esteem, thus, attachment was an intervening variable through which pet type related to one's self-esteem rating. This finding could be explained in part by the previous discussion on children's attachment to pets often viewed as more interactive animals and the evolvement of the attachment relationship between human and animal among high school participants. By the time individuals reach the high school level, they have possibly had a variety of experiences with companion animals, such as the acquisition and care of pets, the loss of a pet, and exposure to some type of animal cruelty. These animal experiences may consciously or even unconsciously influence their attitude toward and attachment to their present companion animals and, consequently, their attitude toward themselves. Another plausible explanation is the assumption that high school students are more advanced socially, emotionally, and cognitively, compared with elementary and middle school children, thus enabling high school students to better understand the complexity of human-animal interactions.

Path analysis was chosen for data analysis because this method is most effective for examining a multidimensional construct such as human-animal relationships. Path analysis is beneficial for estimating the magnitude of linkages between variables while providing information about underlying causal processes. Although the empirical estimates of path coefficients are important in interpretation of results, these statistics must be viewed in conjunction with principles of behavior under investigation, and the credibility of a path analysis model cannot be based on statistical criteria alone but must also be grounded in theory (Bohmestedt & Knoch,

1994). The primary purpose of using path analysis in this study was to assist in the building of a new conceptual framework, rather than to test specific theoretical principles.

This study demonstrated that a new conceptual framework of human-animals relations, based on attachment and self-esteem theory, is theoretically and empirically plausible. Combining key components from both these theoretical frameworks and applying them to the study of human-animal relationships offer promising insight and depth in an effort to better understand these complex relationships. This study examined the relationship between attachment to companion animals and self-esteem in a way unique from previous literature. Although the results of this study indicate that companion animals contribute to the well-being of humans, some questions remain unanswered. Future research would ideally include longitudinal studies following children from elementary school through high school to document developmental changes. The identification of additional intervening variables influencing attachment and self-esteem would broaden the scope of this seemingly complex phenomenon. Comparison of global versus context-specific ratings of self-esteem as related to attachment to companion animals could add insight into the factors influencing this highly debated construct. Finally, including owners of a greater variety of pets in future studies would enable researchers to better understand the unique qualities of human-animal attachment relationships.

References

Abramowitz, R. H., Peterson, A. C., & Schulenberg, J. E. (1984). Changes in self-image during early adolescence. *New Directions for Mental Health Services, 22,* 19-28.

Ainsworth, M. D. S. (1969). Object relations, dependency, and attachment: A theoretical review of the infant-mother relationship. *Child Development, 40*(4), 969-1025.

Ainsworth, M. D. S. (1982). Attachment: Retrospect and prospect: In C. M. Parkes & J. Stevenson-Hinde (Eds.), *The place of attachment in human behavior* (pp. 3-30) New York: Basic Books.

Beck, A. M., & Katcher, A. H. (1983). *Between pets and people: The importance of animal companionship.* New York: G. P. Putnam.

Block, J., & Robins, R. W. (1993). A longitudinal study of consistency and change in self-esteem from early adolescence to early adulthood. *Child Development, 64,* 909-923.

Bohmestedt, G. W., & Knoch, D. (1994). *Statistics for social data analysis.* Itasca, IL: F. E. Peacock.

Bollen, K. A. (1989). *Structural equations with latent variables.* New York: John Wiley.

Bowlby, J. (1969). *Attachment and loss: Vol. 1. Attachment.* New York: Basic Books.

Coopersmith, S. (1967). *The antecedents of self-esteem.* San Francisco: Freeman.

Demo, D. H. (1985). The measurement of self-esteem: Refining our methods. *Journal of Personality and Social Psychology, 48*(6), 1490-1502.

Harlow, H. F., & Zimmerman, R. R. (1959). Affectional responses in the infant monkey. *Science, 130,* 421-432.

Harter, S. (1983). Developmental perspectives on the self-system. In E. M. Hetherington (Ed.), *Handbook of child psychology: Vol. 4. Socialization, personality, and social development* (pp. 275-385). New York: John Wiley.

Holcomb, R., Williams, C. R., & Richards, R. (1985). The elements of attachment: Relationship maintenance and intimacy. *Journal of the Delta Society, 2*(1), 28-34.

Kidd, A. H., & Kidd, R. M. (1985). Children's attitudes toward their pets. *Psychological Reports, 57,* 15-31.

Levinson, B. M. (1972). *Pets and human development.* Springfield, IL: Charles C Thomas.

Melson, G. F. (1988). Availability of and involvement with pets by children: Determinants and correlates. *Anthrozoös, 2*(1), 45-52.

Melson, G. F., & Fogle, A. (1989). Children's ideas about animal young and their care: A reassessment of gender differences in the development of nurturance. *Anthrozoös, 2*(4), 265-273.

Poresky, R. H., Hendrix, C., Mosier, J., & Samuelson, M. (1987). The companion animal bonding scales: Internal reliability and construct validity. *Psychological Reports, 60,* 743-746.

Robin, M., & ten Bensel, R. (1985). Pets and the socialization of children. *Marriage and Family Review, 8,* 63-78.

Rosenberg, M. (1979). *Conceiving the self.* New York: Basic Books.

Rosenberg, M., Schooler, C., Schoenbach, C., & Rosenberg, F. (1995). Global self-esteem and specific self-esteem: Different concepts, different outcomes. *American Sociological Review, 60,* 141-156.

Stevens, L. T. (1990). Attachment to pets among eighth graders. *Anthrozoös, 3*(3), 177-183.

Triebenbacher, S. L. (1994, October). *Children's use of pets as transitional objects: Their role in children's emotional development.* Paper presented at the annual meeting of the Delta Society, New York.

Blind People and Their Dogs 9

An Empirical Study on Changes in Everyday Life,
in Self-Experience, and in Communication

Melanie C. Steffens
Reinhold Bergler

Abstract

Semistructured interviews lasting 2 to 3 hours were conducted with
80 blind people in Germany, 40 of whom had a guide dog. Content
analyses revealed that dependence on others, constant nervous
strain, social problems, and communication problems are the primary everyday stress factors of blind people. Social support and
the support given by a guide dog are some of the coping strategies
that are used in regard to these stress factors. A comparison of the
use of mobility canes with the company of a guide dog indicated
that those blind people who own a dog clearly prefer the animal, at
least in most situations. To a lesser extent, this statement also holds
for a comparison of human chaperones with guide dogs. Blind
guide dog owners feel more independent with their dogs than they
do in the company of a chaperone. Further, these data also indicate that the support provided by the guide dogs to their owners
actually surpasses the initial high hopes held by the owners. Finally, both blind owners and nonowners perceive many benefits
from a guide dog.

Previous research has shown that dogs play a significant role in their owners' lives as well as in society as a whole (e.g., Bergler, 1986; Bergler, 1988). Some examples of this are numerous portrayals of dogs in the arts (e.g., literature, painting, and sculpture), "pet-facilitated psychotherapy" (Bergler, 1988, p. 41), and the role dogs play in the lives of different age groups, especially children and older persons. According to the results of a representative study in Germany, dog ownership is, among many other things, related to social stimulation, companionship, fulfillment of emotional needs, leisure activity, and preventive health care. In addition, service dogs stimulate verbal and nonverbal communication between people in wheelchairs and passersby, according to research using self-report measures (Hart, Hart, & Bergin, 1987) as well as measures of systematic observation (Eddy, Hart, & Boltz, 1988).

Surprisingly few published psychological studies, however, deal with the relationship between blind people and their guide dogs and with the significance these dogs have for blind people. For example, a search of one of the international databases (e.g., PsycLIT) yielded only a few publications that are related to the topic of this pilot study. One publication reported that one of the central factors that contribute to successful mobility training with blind people is their having a guide dog (Gillman & Simon, 1982). Hill and Jacobson (1985) critically compare dog guides with mobility canes to find that in most instances, the dogs are preferred choice. Another publication dealt with the role of matching guide dogs and blind people who fit together well (Robson, 1985). A study in Northern Ireland (Jackson et al., 1994) concluded that blind people who own guide dogs are a selected subgroup of the population of blind people, being younger and healthier and having been visually impaired for a longer time than an average blind person. Blind people owning guide dogs also seem to have higher self-esteem than blind people who do not own guide dogs (Delafield, 1975). In a closely related study, Lambert (1990) addressed the problems and benefits associated with using a guide dog from a theoretical point of view based on psychoanalytical concepts, considering factors such as anxiety, embarrassment, and the dependence-independence conflict that arises in the relationship between a blind person and his or her dog.

In contrast to Lambert's approach, this study asked blind people how their lives are with and without guide dogs. This exploratory, psychological study consisted of open-ended questions asked of 80 blind individuals (40 with guide dogs and 40 without guide dogs) in a 2- to 3-hour interview.

TABLE 9.1 Demographic Characteristics of the Sample ($N = 80$)		
Variable	*Blind People With Dog* *N = 40* *f*	*Blind People Without Dog* *N = 40* *f*
Gender		
Male	17	23
Female	23	17
Civil status		
Single	11	12
Widow/divorced	10	7
Living with partner/married	19	21
Age		
21 to 30 years	4	12
31 to 40 years	7	3
41 to 50 years	11	12
51 to 60 years	8	6
61 to 70 years	9	4
71+ years	1	3

Table 9.1 presents selected characteristics of the sample; 50% of the sample were male, 50% were female, half lived with a partner, and the other half was single. The majority of the sample participants were more than 40 years old.

The participants' responses were recorded verbatim and later evaluated using content-analysis (cf. Lisch & Kriz, 1973, for a comprehensive overview). Questions concerning the importance of a guide dog for coping with everyday problems and for the quality of life of blind people were the focus of the study. This study is intended to determine how blind people perceive their lives and the role of a guide dog in it. Data are presented not on qualities of guide dogs but rather on their owners' perception of their guide dogs' qualities.

Results

There were no gender differences in the data, so all the results reported are collapsed across male and female participants. This chapter is divided into seven results sections: everyday stress factors of blind people, their coping strategies, the comparison of long canes with guide dogs, the comparison of a human guide with a guide dog, the hopes pinned on a guide dog beforehand, the benefits of a guide dog, and the role of the dog in stimulating social contacts.

Common Stress Factors of Blind People

In daily life, blind people are confronted with a multitude of problems that often lead to stress. Strategies are not always available to solve these problems. In the interviews, participants mentioned many problems spontaneously. For this study, each problem or stress factor included was mentioned by at least four people.

Permanent stress factors include dependence, helplessness, loss of spontaneous decision making, nervous strain, the need for concentration, and slowness. Second, there are social problems such as others' prejudice and insufficient social acceptance, problems in finding and making contact, loneliness, and pity by others. Third, blind people experience communicative problems. Because of their loss of visual contact, there is a loss of ability to differentiate between sociopositive and socionegative behavior, a loss of spontaneous sympathetic and antipathetic judgment, and an inability to perceive nonverbal feedback. Last, general uncertainty in orientation in buildings, in traffic, and in strange surroundings was frequently mentioned.

Coping With Everyday Problems

Manifold problems can be handled in various ways: social support provided through family, friends, or employees of social welfare facilities; support given by a guide dog; optimizing behavior by analyzing errors; and communicating with other blind people. A less positive means of handling stressors includes suppression or resignation. These data reveal that forms of resignation are observed only in a minority of blind people interviewed. More typically, a style prevails that can be characterized by actively overcoming problems, by communicating, and by taking social support for granted.

Comparing Long Canes With Guide Dog

A long cane (i.e., a mobility stick) or white stick, along with a multitude of practical aids, is of great significance for blind people. Of all blind

TABLE 9.2	Use of a Guide Dog or a Long Cane by Blind People With and Without Guide Dogs (*N* = 80)	
	Number of Replies as a Percentage	
Using the Mobility/Long Cane	*Blind People With Dogs* *n = 40*	*Blind People Without Dogs* *n = 40*
Using cane	65	95
Not using cane	35	5

people without a guide dog in this sample, 95% use a cane, whereas only 65% of blind people with dogs additionally use a cane to orient themselves, and they do so only in specific situations (see Table 9.2).

According to the responses of blind people in this sample, among the risks associated with long canes are a permanent insecurity despite mobility training, constant high concentration and stress, frequent loss of orientation, and being stigmatized as handicapped. As one participant put it, "I felt ugly and clumsy with a cane—really handicapped, thus I often didn't go out for days on end."

Once a person who is blind has a guide dog, the dog is definitely preferred over a cane. The significant advantages that a guide dog has compared with a long cane include an early warning of obstacles and being led around them, recognizing changes or possible hazards earlier, and a way of moving forward safely even in crowds. Furthermore, the dog provides advantages on strange paths and in strange surroundings and greater speed in moving forward, and the harness can be gripped more firmly and securely than a cane. The interviews showed that the dog is perceived not as a gadget with limited scope but as a partner who enables a blind person to find quicker, safer ways of solving problems.

Comparison of Support to a Blind Person
by a Human Being and by a Guide Dog

Blind people have to learn early in their lives that they cannot survive without help from others; they learn to accept the various forms of social support and take them for granted. Nevertheless, being dependent on others creates strain occasionally on almost half of the respondents (see Table 9.3).

TABLE 9.3   How Blind People Cope With Their Increased Need of Social Support (N = 80)

Being Dependent on Social Support	Number of Replies as a Percentage N = 80
Social support is not regarded as a nuisance and as depressing	58
Social support is regarded as a nuisance and as depressing	23
Depending on the situation, social support is regarded as a nuisance and as depressing	19

TABLE 9.4   Amount of Independence Blind People Feel When Accompanied by Person or Dog (N = 40)

Amount of Independence/Freedom Experienced: "Dog as Helper" Compared With a Person	Number of Replies as a Percentage N = 40
Greater independence and freedom through a dog	55
Greater independence and freedom through a person	10
Amount of independence experienced dependent on situation	35

There are limits to mutual tolerance for blind people and for those who assist them, and conflicts are possible. In our comparison of humans and guide dogs as helpers, we found that guide dogs can prevent such conflicts arising. Of all blind respondents with a dog, 50% prefer to be accompanied by their dogs when they go out. Forty-five percent differ to a greater extent in the specific situation and their own actual requirements; sometimes they prefer the dog, sometimes a person. These preferences stem from the greater freedom that blind people experience through their dogs in comparison with human chaperones (see Table 9.4).

The reasons for this are varied and show how much a guide dog increases a blind person's subjective feeling of freedom. With the dog, there is no need to justify oneself, no criticism. The dog is constantly present and available; there is no need to ask for everything. The dog is reported to be more reliable in guiding and is perceived to truly enjoy guiding the person.

A blind person cannot and does not want to do without help from other human beings; this is particularly true in all places that ban dogs and in conjunction with verbal communication and the purchase of certain products such as clothes. Even though guide dogs are allowed in grocery stores and government offices (as required by federal laws in Germany), many blind people report that conflicts have arisen when they tried to enter such places in the company of their guide dogs.

Hopes Placed on a Guide Dog

Before they had their first guide dog, 90% of all blind people pinned extremely positive hopes on the dog. These expectations, however, were surpassed in 85% of all cases. Blind people had underestimated the amount of actual help and support, the amount of independence they achieved with the aid of the dog, and the amount of safe orientation in strange surroundings. In addition, the dog's significance as a friend and the extent that the dog facilitated contact with other people were underestimated. A good guide dog is generally a positive surprise for the blind person. The dog is supplementary to the technical aids already available, and, more important, it reduces dependency and increases quality of life.

Benefits of a Guide Dog

Analysis of the significance of guide dogs for blind people compared with corresponding data of a representative random sample of (nonguide) dog owners (see Bergler, 1988) indicates that the perceived and expected benefits of a guide dog are more differentiated for all blind people, no matter whether they actually own a dog or not. There are stronger emotional ties between blind people and their dogs than in an average population of dog owners (see Table 9.5).

The Guide Dog as a Social Stimulant

Almost all respondents indicated that touching, playing with, and communicating with their dogs are of key importance to them. The advantages of guide dogs include more contacts with other people, less tension and

TABLE 9.5   Benefits of Guide Dogs as Seen by Blind People (N = 80)

The Benefit Profile of a Guide Dog: Spontaneous Replies	Number of Replies as a Percentage (Several Answers Possible) N = 80
Feeling and returning affection, love, tenderness	98
Dog as a comrade and faithful partner	88
Playing together with dog	88
Guard against being alone and loneliness	68
More frequent and more intensive contacts with other people	68
Increased independence, not having to rely on help from others	68
Increased mobility and flexibility	66
Increased safety: dog as a protector	51
Increased safety amid traffic	48
Being safely guided and led around obstacles	39
Less strain on nerves due to quiet, relaxed walking	18
Dog as a cuddly object to fondle	15
Better orientation in strange surroundings	10
Alleviating orientation fears	10
Promoting health and fitness and structuring daily routine	7

strain, and more relaxed walking leading to increased fitness and structuring of the activities of daily life. Most blind people experience or expect increased independence and mobility with their guide dogs, and they feel safer with their dogs. When the dogs are not "in service," the respondents reported that they and the dogs enjoyed playing together.

For blind people, guide dogs are a help in judging their social environment and establishing and deepening contact with other people. The majority (88%) of the respondents stated that it is easier to get to know people with the dogs present. For nearly 80% of the sample, dogs are often the topic of conversation with others; for 15%, relatively often; and for 7%, rarely the topic of conversation.

Conclusions

Statistical comparisons of responses between dog owners and non-owners were not possible because of the structure of this exploratory study. The preponderance of evidence, however, leads us to conclude that for 95% of the blind individuals sampled with a guide dog, life would not be conceivable without the dog. For a blind person with a dog, the amount of everyday stress is reduced and the amount of everyday pleasures is increased. Additional research with a refined methodological approach to assessing quality of life markers is the next appropriate step in building the knowledge base in this area of study.

References

Bergler, R. (1986). *Mensch und Hund: Psychologie einer Beziehung* [Human and dog: The psychology of a relationship]. Cologne, Germany: Agrippa.

Bergler, R. (1988). *Man and dog: The psychology of a relationship.* Oxford, UK: Blackwell Scientific.

Delafield, G. (1975). *Self-perception and the effects of mobility training.* Unpublished doctoral dissertation, University of Nottingham, Nottingham, UK.

Eddy, J., Hart, L. A., & Boltz, R. P. (1988). The effects of service dogs on social acknowledgments of people in wheelchairs. *Journal of Psychology, 122,* 39-45.

Gillman, A. E., & Simon, E. P. (1982). A summary of a two-part mobility study. *International Journal of Rehabilitation Research, 5,* 394.

Hart, L. A., Hart, B. L., & Bergin, B. (1987). Socializing effects of service dogs for people with disabilities. *Anthrozoös, 1,* 41-44.

Hill, E. W., & Jacobson, W. H. (1985). Controversial issues in orientation and mobility: Then and now. *Education of the Visually Handicapped, 17,* 59-70.

Jackson, A. J., Murphy, P. J., Dusoir, T., Dusoir, H., Murdock, A., & Morrison, E. (1994). Ophthalmic, health and social profile of guide dog owners in Northern Ireland. *Ophthalmic and Physiological Optics, 14,* 371-377.

Lambert, R. M. (1990). Some thoughts about acquiring and learning to use a dog guide. *Review, 22,* 151-158.

Lisch, R., & Kriz, J. (1973). *Grundlagen und Modelle der Inhaltsanalyse* [Foundations and models of content analysis]. Reinbek, Germany: Rowohlt.

Robson, H. (1985). Dog guide and blind person: The matching process. *Journal of Visual Impairment and Blindness, 79,* 356.

PART IV

Quality of Life Outcomes: The Relevance of Animals to Health and Disease

Cindy C. Wilson
Dennis C. Turner

Cardiovascular patients' satisfaction with outcomes of their care is often related to QL issues, for example, how well they maintain their physical, mental, and cognitive functions and their role with family and friends, at home, at work, and in the larger community to which they belong. This area of research has been fertile for QL markers and HAI. Indeed, it offers the greatest opportunity worldwide to integrate HAI/QL questions in the context of major population studies. In this section, Jennings et al. suggest that more research is needed to determine if pet ownership is simply cardioprotective or whether attributes of pet ownership account for the positive QL effects. McNicholas and Collis apply that concept by examining representation of Type A individuals in pet owners and find that this trait does not explain the association between ownership and health advantages. Friedmann and Thomas once again evaluate the role of HAI as a means of social support for coronary artery disease patients in the Cardiac Arrhythmia Suppression Trial (CAST). They find that pet ownership and social support are related to survival among these patients.

In a different mode, Batson et al. assess the impact of a therapy dog on communication problems and associated stress levels in patients with Alzheimer's and find that although there was a reduction in physiological markers of stress and that communication behaviors tended to improve, the sample size limited the usefulness of the data. The tendency to minimize communication stress, however, as shown by the data, is promising and warrants further study.

Animals and Cardiovascular Health 10

Garry L. R. Jennings
Christopher M. Reid
Irene Christy
Janis Jennings
Warwick P. Anderson
Anthony Dart

Abstract

The potential relationship between pet ownership and cardiovascular disease is intriguing. This chapter provides an overview of several studies that contribute to that line of reasoning as a means of identifying areas of needed research. Cardiovascular risk factors were examined in 5,741 healthy participants attending a screening service. Pet owners had significantly lower systolic blood pressure and plasma triglycerides than nonowners. There were also significantly lower cholesterol values in men but not in women. Systolic blood pressure and triglyceride differences were seen only in women over age 40. Differences in plasma triglycerides and sys-

AUTHORS' NOTE: We greatly acknowledge the support of the staff of the Baker Medical Research Institute Risk Reduction Clinic established by the Rotary Club of Melbourne and funded by the National Mutual Life Association Ltd. We also are grateful for the support of Petcare Information and Advisory Service for the projects conducted at the Baker Institute. We are particularly grateful to Sally Kaye, R.N., who collected data for the case control study.

tolic blood pressure were relatively modest, averaging in men 13% and 2%, respectively. Coupled with the high frequency of ownership of pets in the community, these decreases are considered to be large enough to be important to public health.

Associations such as these are open to various interpretations and do not prove that animal companionship per se lowers cardiovascular risk factors. It is more likely that other attributes, more common in pet owners, account for the relationship. The socioeconomic profile of pet owners and non-pet owners in the sample appeared similar, and the lower risk factor levels were not due to smoking, body weight, or dietary differences. Pet owners did exercise more regularly.

If pet owners have lower levels of cardiovascular risk, then it might be anticipated that cardiovascular disease rates and outcomes would differ from members of the community who do not have animal companions. To examine this, a case control study comparing the rates of pet ownership among participants with newly diagnosed angina and matched controls is being conducted.

To examine the community and cost implications of the putatively lower rates of cardiovascular disease risk factors requires a broader approach. A recent representative national survey of the Australian population found that dog owners had 8% fewer doctor visits in the previous year than non-dog owners. Cat owners had 12% fewer attendances than non-cat owners. This was reflected in lower rates of medication use for high blood pressure, cholesterol, sleeping difficulties, or heart problems.

Cardiovascular diseases, which include coronary heart disease and stroke, are the cause of almost half of all deaths in developed countries, and they are increasing dramatically in other countries with emerging economies. The changes in incidence in cardiovascular disease in various communities suggest that to a large extent, the earlier cardiovascular deaths are preventable. Several countries, including the United States and Australia, experienced a substantial drop in cardiovascular deaths during the past 20 years. About one third of the decrease can be attributed to improvements in medical treatment, but the remainder is either unexplained or due to changes in risk factors that predisposed to atherosclerosis, the underlying cause of most cardiovascular disease. The major known risk factors include smoking, high blood pressure, and high blood cholesterol. Others are physical inactivity, diabetes, obesity, and other metabolic disorders. Psychological stress is less well established as a risk factor for atherosclerosis but may be a precipitant of clinical events in individuals who may have coronary heart disease. The precise contribution of all known risk factors to cardiovascular disease is not really known, but they may account for one half. Clearly, it is likely that other factors are influencing rates of heart disease that are not yet considered as major risk factors. In this light, it is of interest to examine the proposition that close relationship to companion animals may be associated with lower risk of cardiovascular disease.

Pet Ownership and Risk Factors for Cardiovascular Disease

Initial interest in this question was stimulated by examination of the risk factor profile among pet owners and non-pet owners attending a free screening clinic at the Baker Medical Research Institute (Anderson, Reid, & Jennings., 1992). Of 5,741 participants attending during a 3-year period, 784 were pet owners and 4,957 nonowners. The risk factor profile of the attendees was similar to that of a randomly selected population of Australians participating in a national risk prevalence study, thus indicating that these data appear representative of the general population. There were two parts to the assessment. A self-assessment questionnaire included questions on smoking habits, alcohol intake, diabetes, dietary and exercise habits, family history of heart disease, and age. Objective measurements performed at the time of visit included body weight, blood pressure, and cholesterol and triglyceride levels. Participants also completed a brief questionnaire on pet ownership. The study included persons between 20 and 60 years of age.

Pet owners had significantly lower systolic blood pressure and plasma triglycerides than nonowners (Figures 10.1 and 10.2). Male pet owners had significantly lower systolic but not diastolic blood pressure than nonowners and significantly lower plasma triglyceride levels and plasma cholesterol levels. Systolic but not diastolic pressure was significantly lower in female pet owners older than 40 years, and plasma triglycerides tended to be lower. Pet owners and non-pet owners, however, did not differ in body mass index, socioeconomic indicators, or smoking habits. Pet owners exercised significantly more than nonowners. Dietary factors that were

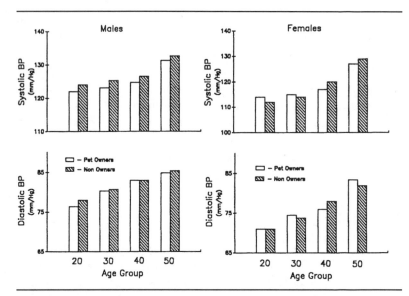

Figure 10.1. Systolic and Diastolic Blood Pressure Levels for Male and Female Participants on the Basis of Pet Ownership

SOURCE: From Anderson, W. P., Reid, C. M., and Jennings, G. L., *Pet Ownership and Risk Factors for Cardiovascular Disease*, Medical Journal of Australia, 1992; 157:298-301. © Copyright 1992. The Medical Journal of Australia. by Reproduced with permission.

NOTE: Age groups 20 through 50 represent 20-29 years, 30-39 years, 40-49 years, and 50-59 years.

different between pet owners and nonowners might have been expected to have the opposite effect on cardiovascular risk factors. For example, owners ate more meat and take-out foods.

These findings raise the possibility that pet ownership reduces cardiovascular risk factors. On the other hand, these findings may be a marker of other undefined characteristics of those who owned pets that led to lower levels of blood pressure and lipids, and the association was not causal. There were no obvious biases in the population study, however, and the lower levels of accepted risk factors for cardiovascular disease was not explicable on the basis of cigarette smoking, diet, body mass index, or socioeconomic profile. Higher exercise levels may have been important in explaining some of the findings, although there was no evidence from this survey that the results were any different for dog owners than for those having other pets such as fish, for which a relationship to exercise habits is intuitively less obvious.

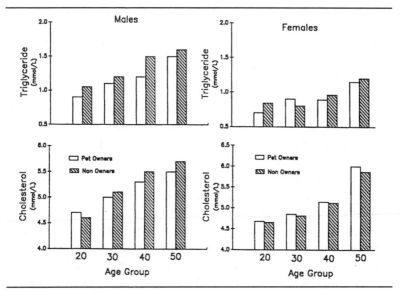

Figure 10.2. Cholesterol and Triglyceride Levels for Male and Female Participants on the Basis of Pet Ownership
SOURCE: SOURCE: From Anderson, W. P., Reid, C. M., and Jennings, G. L., *Pet Ownership and Risk Factors for Cardiovascular Disease*, Medical Journal of Australia, 1992; 157:298-301. © Copyright 1992. The Medical Journal of Australia. by Reproduced with permission.
NOTE: Age groups 20 through 50 represent 20-29 years, 30-39 years, 40-49 years, and 50-59 years.

The differences in risk factors that were observed were relatively modest. In men, triglyceride levels were 13% lower in pet owners, and cholesterol levels were 2% lower. Given the high rate of pet ownership in the community and the prevalence of cardiovascular disease, however, they cannot be dismissed as unimportant. Small reductions in total cholesterol level are associated with quite marked reductions in cardiovascular morbidity and mortality in major treatment trials. The small difference in systolic blood pressure seen between male pet owners and nonowners is similar to those reported for a number of other nonpharmacological means of lowering blood pressure that have become accepted modalities for treatment in hypertension (Jennings, 1990). These results were consistent with previous evidence that acute physical intervention with pets is associated with acute lowering of blood pressure (Katcher, 1981; Messent, 1983; Serpell, 1990). These results extended this evidence into the chronic setting, however, and the plasma lipids results were novel.

Pet Ownership and Incidence of Angina

🐾 An association of pet ownership with lower levels of cardiovascular risk factors is potentially of major clinical importance, To confirm that these changes are significant to quality of life and health, however, it is necessary to show that the lower levels of risk factors in pet owners is carried through to a lower incidence of clinical disease. A case control study was undertaken to examine this question. Because there is always the possibility that those who have already developed coronary heart disease are more likely to be pet owners, the study was confined to newly diagnosed participants with angina and obtained information about pet ownership at the time of their diagnosis and before they had had an opportunity to make any lifestyle changes.

A chest pain questionnaire was administered to participants attending a health screening facility recruited by advertisement from the community. The purpose of the overall project was to examine a relationship between dietary intake and subsequent development of cancer, so there was no reason to consider that biases related to a particular interest in pets might have affected the population under study. Participants whose responses to the chest pain questionnaire indicated the possibility of angina were then assessed more thoroughly. Electrocardiographic monitoring during an exercise test identified participants displaying both symptoms of typical angina and ST segment depression during exercise who subsequently met the criteria for entry to the study. Although these were the defining criteria for entry, two thirds of the group identified in this way subsequently had coronary angiography, and many have since had coronary artery bypass grafting or coronary angioplasty. Controls were selected from the same community survey; controls were matched to each case for gender, age, and cholesterol level. In an initial analysis, there was clear underrepresentation of pet owners among males with angina compared with controls (Table 10.1). Whereas 43% of cases owned pets, the proportion owning pets among controls was 70% ($p < 0.01$). This study is continuing, and the study population has subsequently been increased. The final results will include data from more than 50 cases with angina, with 2 matched controls per case to more accurately define the expected rate of pet ownership among healthy participants.

TABLE 10.1   Frequency of Pet Ownership Among Cases With
Newly Diagnosed Angina (CHD) and Controls
Matched for Gender, Age, and Cholesterol

| | Percentage of Pet Owners | | |
	All	Males	Females
CHD	55	43	75
Control	71	70	71
	$p < 0.05$	$p < 0.01$	

Implications of an Association Between Pet Ownership and Cardiovascular Health and Health Costs

In November 1994, the Australian People and Pet Survey was conducted to provide a nationwide representative survey to evaluate health benefits associated with pet ownership (McHarg, Baldock, Headey, & Robinson, 1995). A national stratified probability sample of 1,011 people were interviewed by telephone. The sampling size and procedures followed a model established by the surveying organization (The Roy Morgan Research Centre) for election surveys. The initial respondent to the telephone call was first asked if the household had a pet and if so, what type. If the answer was positive, the interviewer asked to interview the main caregiver of the dog. If there was no dog, the interviewer requested to speak to the primary caregiver of the first pet mentioned. Of the total number of households, 60% had pets. In the remaining 40% of the sample, interviews were conducted on pet-related issues and on health issues. Forty percent of households owned one or more dogs, 27% owned cats, and less than 15% owned other types of pets. These estimates are consistent with those from previous surveys.

Two specific questions were included to assess implications of pet ownership for use of health services. The first question was, "During the last year, how many times would you say that you have been to the doctor—I mean any sort of doctor, your family doctor or specialists. About how many times?" The second query was, "I would like to ask you a few questions about any medicine that you may be taking at present. Are you taking medication, either tablets or liquid, for any of the following conditions: high blood pressure, high cholesterol, sleeping difficulties, a heart problem?" Other questions were included to assess exercise levels, frequency of petting or grooming the animal, level of social networks, and perceived closeness to the pet. Statistical procedures were used to control for gender, age, and other factors known to influence use of health care services. As in similar surveys, this was necessary because more women were pet carers than men, and older people had fewer pets, particularly dogs, than did younger people.

The results indicated that dog and cat owners visited the doctor in the past year less frequently than nonowners and were less likely to be taking medication for heart problems, high blood pressure, high cholesterol, or sleeping difficulties. The average number of doctor visits per year among nonowners was five. Significantly lower rates were observed in those owning a dog or cat or a cat alone ($p < 0.05$). There was a trend toward lower number of doctor visits among those owning only a dog or both dog and cat. Of non-pet owners, 19% were taking one or other of the specified medications. Lower rates were observed in all categories owning pets with statistically significant reductions, $p < 0.01$, in those owning dog or cat (12%), dog alone (11%), or dog and cat (11%). A number of subgroups were examined according to gender and age (i.e., less than 25, 25 to 54, or over 55). All gender-age groups except men aged 25 to 54 showed fewer numbers of doctor visits in the last year than nonowners. Among older men and women, use of medication also appeared to be considerably less among pet owners. Because of the small subsample sizes, none of these differences were significant.

There was some evidence that having a pet was associated with better social networks and reduced loneliness. Of pet owners, 58% said they made friends through owning pets. Similarly, 62% of owners said that having a pet around when people were around or visited made conversation easier and helped create a friendly atmosphere. The majority of owners (79%) found it comforting to be with their pets when things went wrong, and 91% said they felt very close to their pets, almost as many who felt very close to their families. Nonpartnered people who reported feeling close to their dogs made significantly fewer doctor visits and took less medication than nonpartnered people who were not close to their dogs. There was no evidence that those owning multiple animals fared better in measures of health or social networks than those with a single animal. These findings have led Headey (1995) to propose a mechanism whereby owning a dog might improve health through both increasing exercise levels, an established measure for reducing cardiovascular risk, and reducing loneliness. Although loneliness has not been established as a cardinal risk factor for cardiovascular disease, it has been advocated as a possible aggravating factor in a wide range of human disease.

An economic analysis of the above results sought to establish the actual cost of doctor visits and medication use in a number of ways (Anderson, Headey, & Newby, 1995). This analysis included average *per capita* benefits, average *per capita* prescription costs, and the costs of general practitioner visits. On the basis of the Australian Department of Human Services and Health (1995) *Statistical Overview, 1993-94* the value of *per capita* medical benefits in that year for males was $243.84; for females, $358.46; for a total of $301.36. According to the (1991) 1989-1990 Australian Bureau of Statistics health survey, adult males aged between 25 to 64 years have an annual rate of visits to their doctors of 5.21, adult females have a rate if 8.21, for an overall visitation rate of 6.61. The total average cost including government and patient contributions per prescription in 1993-1994 was $16.62; 114.02 million prescriptions were processed in Australia. If there is indeed a causal relationship between pet ownership and health, three categories of savings are plausible: savings due to fewer doctors visits, savings due to lower consumption of medications, and savings due to lower rates of hospitalization. It is possible from these data to construct a hypothetical situation in which there are no pets and to estimate the health savings from the present levels of pet ownership. The annual savings (in Australian dollars) for main caregivers were calculated as follows:

Savings from GP visits:
2.7 million × 0.4 fewer doctor
visits × $24.30 per visit = $26.244 million

Savings on pharmaceuticals:
2.7 million × 0.4 × 0.9 probability of getting
prescription × $19.40 per script = $18.856 million

Savings on hospitalization:
2.7 million × 0.4 × 0.033 probability of being hospitalized
after a GP visit × $2,800 cost of the average 2-day
hospitalization = $99.792 million

Total: $144.892 million

Additional savings could be assumed if other family members also gained some of the benefits from pet ownership. Although the differences in levels of risk factors for cardiovascular disease observed in this risk screening survey were small, they could, if directly due to the presence of a close relationship to pets, provide health benefits to a larger community. This potential benefit occurs because of the high prevalence of cardiovascular disease and its risk factors in the community and the high percentage of pet ownership households in Australia and similar countries.

Conclusion

These data provide presumptive evidence of a link between animal companionship and cardiovascular disease. It would be premature to conclude that measures that seek to increase the level of pet ownership in the community would result in further lowering of cardiovascular disease rates. The results, however, prompt further research in this area as potentially fruitful. The main limitation of the studies presented is that they describe correlations that may be merely fortuitous. A large number of patients, however, were surveyed with detailed documentation of their cardiovascular risk status, and careful attention was paid to the elimination of bias in the study designs. A surprising tendency for several known risk factors for cardiovascular disease to be lower in pet owners and for the use of health services by pet owners to be consistently lower was found. The nature of these studies does not allow us to attribute the differences necessarily to pet ownership itself because it is uncertain that these studies include comparable samples for the general population. There was evidence, however, that the socioeconomic profile and cardiovascular risk factor profile were representative of the general population. Thus, the hypothesis that pet ownership lowers cardiovascular disease rates should be tested in controlled perspective studies.

References

Anderson, W., Headey, B., & Newby, J. (1995). *Health costs savings: The impact of pets on Australian health budgets.* Melbourne, Victoria, Australia: Petcare Information and Advisory Service.

Anderson, W. P., Reid, C. M., & Jennings, G. L. (1992). Pet ownership and risk factors for cardiovascular disease. *Medical Journal of Australia, 157,* 298-301.

Australian Bureau of Statistics. (1991, August). *National health survey: Summary of results 1989-1990* (No. 4364.0). Canberra, Australian Capital Territory: Author.

Australian Department of Human Services and Health. (1995). *Statistical overview 1993-94.* Canberra, Australian Capital Territory: AGPS.

Headey, B. (1995). *Health benefits of pets: Results from the Australian people and pets survey.* Melbourne, Victoria, Australia: Petcare Information and Advisory Service.

Jennings, G. L. (1990). Prospects for the non-pharmacological control of hypertension. In J. K. McNeil, R. W. F. King, G. L. Jennings, & J. W. Powles (Eds.), *A textbook of preventive medicine* (pp. 133-145). Melbourne, Victoria, Australia: Edward Arnold.

Katcher, A. H. (1981). Interactions between people and their pets: Form and function. In B. Fogle (Ed.), *Interrelations between people and pets* (pp. 41-67). Springfield, IL: Charles C Thomas.

McHarg, M., Baldock, C., Headey, B., & Robinson, A. (1995). *National people and pets survey.* Sydney, New South Wales, Australia: Urban Animal Management Coalition.

Messent, P. R. (1983). A review of recent developments in human-companion animal studies. *California Veterinarian, 5,* 26-50.

Serpell, J. A. (1990). Evidence for long-term effects of pet ownership on human health. In I. H. Berger (Ed.), *Pets, benefits and practice* (pp. 1-7). London: BVA.

Could Type A (Coronary Prone) Personality Explain the Association Between Pet Ownership and Health? 11

June McNicholas
Glyn M. Collis

Abstract

Three classes of explanation are identified for the reported associations between pet ownership and advantages for human health: direct causal effects of pet ownership; indirect causal effects mediated, for example, by the influence of pets on the network of human social contacts; and noncausal effects whereby some factor(s) influence both health and the propensity to own a pet. This study investigates Type A personality as a candidate factor underlying a noncausal explanation. Our hypothesis is that people exhibiting high levels of Type A behavior may be less likely to own a pet because their elevated levels of hostility and impatience and that their hard-driving, ambitious, and hectic lifestyles may not dispose them toward pet ownership. Because Type A behavior is associated with increased risk of stress-related illness, including coronary heart disease, if it were found that Type A personalities were underrepresented among pet owners, this would have impor-

AUTHORS' NOTE: During the preparation of this chapter, we were in receipt of financial support from the Waltham Centre for Pet Nutrition. June McNicholas is a Waltham Research Fellow.

tant implications for studies reporting health advantages accruing to pet owners because people electing to own pets could be a population already at lower risk of stress-related illness. A brief Type A scale (Järvikoski & Härkäpää, 1987) was administered to 541 adult participants, from whom information was also collected on pet ownership and various demographic variables. Against expectation, pet owners had higher Type A scores than nonowners. These higher scores may reflect the busy-energetic-active aspect of the Type A trait, rather than the ambitious-competitive-impatient aspect, but the data rule out a noncausal explanation for health advantage based on this factor.

Introduction

🐾 Recent studies have demonstrated an association between pet ownership and advantages for physical and psychological health. For example, one large-scale study conducted in a cardiovascular risk screening clinic in Australia reported an association between pet ownership and lower levels of risk factors for cardiovascular disease (Anderson, Reid, & Jennings, 1992). Levels of plasma triglycerides, cholesterol, and systolic blood pressure were found to be lower in pet owners, especially among males. These findings could not be explained by differences in age, socioeconomic background, smoking, alcohol consumption, or dietary habits. In addition to findings of lower heart rate and blood pressure as an immediate consequence of contact with animals (Friedmann, Katcher, Thomas, Lynch, & Messent, 1983) are reports that pet ownership is associated with better recovery from myocardial infarction (Friedmann, Katcher, Lynch, & Thomas, 1980) and that the acquisition of pets is associated with a lower incidence of minor physical ailments and higher ratings of psychological well-being (Serpell, 1991).

Such findings have received considerable publicity and have quickly resulted in a widespread lay belief that pets are good for health. As yet, little is known about how such health benefits accrue to pet owners or, indeed, if they are truly attributable to pet ownership.

Three broad classes of mechanisms have been proposed to explain the association between pet ownership and health. It has been suggested that all three classes should be further investigated empirically (McNicholas, Collis, & Morley, 1995). These classes of mechanisms are depicted in

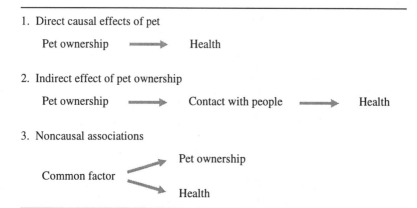

1. Direct causal effects of pet

    Pet ownership   ⟶   Health

2. Indirect effect of pet ownership

    Pet ownership   ⟶   Contact with people   ⟶   Health

3. Noncausal associations

    Common factor ⟨   Pet ownership

                         Health

Figure 11.1. Three Classes of Explanation for the Association Between Pet Ownership and Advantages for Health

Figure 11.1. The first class of mechanism is a direct causal effect of pet ownership on health. For example, where the pet is regarded as a significant relationship by the owner, it may be perceived as providing social support that could alleviate adverse responses to stress. This proposal is examined in Chapter 6. In the second class of mechanism, pet ownership may exert an indirect effect by enhancing their owners' social networks of human contacts. Pets, particularly dogs, are powerful catalysts for human social interactions (McNicholas, Collis, Morley, & Lane, 1993; Messent, 1983). For many owners, these casual meetings become regular and established joint recreational activity and interest. Some of the contacts made through pets become friendships that extend beyond the shared interest in animals into non-pet-centered activities. In this model, the health benefits are derived from the companionship, support, and involvement in an enhanced network of human social contacts.

In the third class of mechanism, the association between pet ownership and health may be noncausal in nature (i.e., there may be some other factor(s) that can explain both health advantages and the propensity to own a pet). As yet, there appears to be no research that has demonstrated significant differences between pet owners and nonowners in ways that could also explain health benefits. Nonetheless, this particular class of explanation should be investigated most thoroughly if the proposal that pet ownership is beneficial to health is accepted. This study is an investigation of one such factor (i.e., Type A personality) that could explain the association between pet ownership and health in noncausal terms.

What Is Type A personality?

Initially, the Type A construct was first proposed by Friedman & Rosenman (1974) to describe behaviors of persons they identified as overrepresented in their cardiology practice. These patients displayed behavior characterized by a high sense of competition, a desire for recognition and achievement, a sense of urgency and impatience, together with a tendency toward hostility and aggression.

Since the identification of Type A behavior, numerous studies have been conducted in an attempt to validate it as a construct and examine its predictive validity as a coronary risk factor. To date, the evidence is somewhat unclear whether Type A behavior as a whole truly predicts elevated risks for coronary heart disease or whether it may have wider implications for risk of various illnesses, especially stress-related illness (Rime, Ucros, Bestgen, & Jeanjean, 1989). A recent Finnish study found that people with high scores on a Type A scale reported severe angina pectoris symptoms more frequently than did people with low scores on the Type A scale, with high-scoring male participants also reporting more severe chest pain indicative of possible myocardial infarction (Järvikoski & Härkäpää, 1987).

In this study, there is less concern with the validity of its predictive power for coronary heart disease per se than the identification of behavior patterns that may influence both motivation to own a pet and predisposition toward a range of stress-related illnesses. A measure of Type A behavior/personality was believed to fulfill these criteria.

The motivation behind selecting Type A behavior as a possible noncausal factor to link pet ownership and health is based on Type A personalities' exhibition of particular behaviors and attitudes that are believed to elevate their risks for stress-related illness, including coronary heart disease. These same behaviors and attitudes may also make them less likely to own pets. Studies should investigate whether high-risk populations are underrepresented among pet owners. It is plausible that Type A personalities may not find pet ownership compatible with their hard-driving, ambitious, and materialist lifestyles. Thus, people who score highly on a Type A personality questionnaire would be underrepresented as pet owners.

Method

The sample consisted of 541 employees of a city council in the English Midlands who responded to a Healthy Living Survey arranged by the council for its employees. Although encouraged by the council, participation in the survey was voluntary, and returns were anonymous. There were 237 males and 301 females in the sample (three respondents did not indicate their sex). The age of the participants ranged from 17 to 65 years and was distributed as follows: 44 (8%) 17 to 25 years, 118 (22%) 26 to 35 years, 191 (35%) 36 to 45 years, 135 (25%) 46 to 55 years, and 52 (10%) 56 to 65 years. One respondent did not indicate her age. A broad range of occupational grades and types was represented.

The Healthy Living Survey was a questionnaire designed specifically for this study to complement an existing Healthy Lifestyle Campaign currently operating by the city council for its employees. It included a series of questions on demographic variables (age, employment grade or post, marital status, and children), health (major illness in the last 2 years), self-perceived current health (poor, a few problems, fair, good, or excellent), self-perceived physical fitness (poor, fair, good, or excellent), and lifestyle choices (smoking, alcohol consumption, and membership of clubs and societies). Questions about pet ownership were included among the other questions on demographic details. Respondents were asked to indicate the number of pets in their household under the headings cats, dogs, birds, fish, and others or to tick (i.e., check) a box marked none. Respondents with one or more pets in their household were also asked if they considered any of the pets as particularly belonging to them. Our aim for the inclusion of this question was to identify if people scoring high on the Type A scale were pet owners by choice or merely by virtue of sharing a household with a pet belonging to another family member. Finally, the survey included the 15-item Type A personality scale described by Järvikoski and Härkäpää (1987) to have reasonable internal consistency and good predictive validity. The decision to use this scale was based on its recent use on a large sample of 3,221 state employees in Finland. Because the scale was administered in its English form, it was not piloted further for this study and only a few minor changes in wording were made to make it more acceptable to our British sample.

Results

As in the original study by Järvikoski and Härkäpää (1987), one item in the Type A scale (their question 1) correlated very weakly with the sum of the other items and was dropped from the scale. With the remaining 14 items, the scale was found to have reasonably satisfactory internal consistency (Cronbach's alpha = 0.654), which compares well with the 0.69 reported by Järvikoski and Härkäpää. Although this is not as high as could be desirable, it is comparable with the widely used Framingham Scale (Haynes, Feinleib, & Levine, 1978). Each participant's Overall Type A Score represents an average across 14 items, each on a 5-point scale from 1 to 5. For the 529 of the 541 participants who gave complete data on the Type A scale, the mean score was 3.208, standard deviation 0.497, median 3.214, and range 1.714 to 4.786.

Because animals from a wide range of species are kept as pets, and these are likely to vary in their role for their owners, the first comparison is between the following three groups: (1) participants whose household included one or more cats and/or dogs (as prototypical pet species), with or without other species; (2) participants who had pets of other species but not cats or dog; (3) participants who had no pets of any species. Of the 541 participants, 236 (43%) reported having no pets at all, 214 (40%) reported having a cat and/or a dog with or without other species, and 91 (17%) reported having other species but not a cat or dog. The other species included fish, lizards, birds, guinea pigs, hamsters, gerbils, chipmunks, chinchillas, foxes, geese, goats, tortoises, stick insects, rats, and mice.

The two sexes were more or less equally represented among these three pet ownership groups, χ^2 (2, $N = 538$) = 4.16, $p = .125$, with a slight tendency for a higher proportion of males to be nonowners. There was significant variation in the pet ownership groups among the five age groups, χ^2 (8, $N = 540$) = 18.68, $p = .017$, with respondents aged 56 to 65 years having a higher than average incidence of nonowners (62%) and a lower than average incidence of cat/dog owners (23%).

A three-way analysis of variance on the Overall Type A Scores comparing the three groups, with age and sex as background factors, showed a significant main effect of pet ownership group, F (2, 496) = 5.36, $p = .005$. The mean Type A scores were 3.224 for the cat/dog owners ($n = 206$), 3.288 for the owners of other species ($n = 88$), and 3.067 for the nonowners ($n = 232$). Pairwise comparisons using Tukey's HSD method showed both that the cat/dog owners differed from the nonowners ($p = .023$) and that the owners of other species also differed from nonowners ($p = .020$). These findings are illustrated in Figure 11.2. The main effect of age was marginally significant, F (4, 496) = 2.37, $p = .052$, an effect that was almost entirely due to a quadratic trend, F (1, 496) = 7.25, $p = .007$. Mean Overall

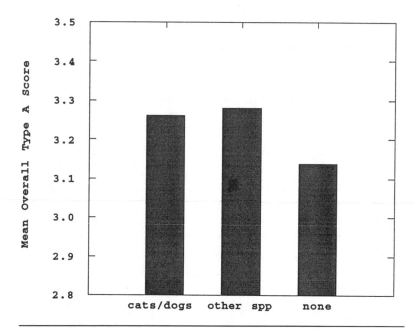

Figure 11.2.   Mean Overall Type A Score by Pet Ownership Group

Type A scores rose from 3.164 in the 17- to 25-year-olds, peaking at 3.282 in both the 26 to 35 and 36 to 45 groups, and dropping to 2.997 in the 56- to 65-year-olds. No other main effects or interactions were statistically significant at $\alpha = 0.05$.

These results indicate that one could not reasonably account for the reported health advantages among pet owners by an underrepresentation of Type A personalities among pet owners because the differences, although small, are statistically significant in a direction opposite to that predicted by the hypothesis.

Although cats and dogs are both prototypical pet species, they are different in character and in relation to their owners. Therefore, the cat/dog owners (pet-owning group 1 as described above) were divided into three subgroups: (a) participants who owned dogs but not cats ($n = 90$), (b) participants who owned cats but not dogs ($n = 85$), and (c) participants who owned both dogs and cats ($n = 32$). In all three subgroups, some participants owned other species, too. A one-factor analysis of variance comparing the three subgroups showed no evidence of differences among their Overall Type A scores, F (2, 204) = 1.38, $p > .25$; means 3.202, 3.321, 3.257 respectively). The smaller number of cases in these subgroups creates a less powerful analysis than the previous analysis of variance, but the tiny differences between the means confirm the absence of important differences. A full three-factor Subgroup x Age x Sex analysis could not be done because of the presence of empty cells, but an analysis was done that showed that a subgroup effect was not simply suppressed by main effects of age or sex.

In surveys of pet ownership, respondents are likely to indicate that they are pet owners on the basis that there are animals in their households. The direct effects model, however, implies that health advantages are most likely to accrue if the pet actually belongs, in some sense, to the respondent, rather than to one or more other persons in the household. Similarly, it was anticipated that Type A personality would be more likely to be under-represented among those participants who reported that a pet was especially regarded as their own pet. Therefore, for pet-owning participants in groups 1 and 2 (cat/dog owners and other species owners), overall Type A scores between participants who answered positively when asked to identify if one or more pets were specifically "yours" were compared with those who answered negatively to this question. A three-factor analysis of variance (Yours/Not Yours x Age x Sex) showed no significant main effects or interactions.

Regarding the main finding (i.e., that overall Type A scores are higher among pet owners than among nonowners), it is possible that this does not apply to the full range of Type A characteristics. For example, it was expected that the aggressively competitive aspects of the Type A personality would not fit well with a pet-owning lifestyle. The component of the Type A concept, however, that emphasizes a busy and energetic lifestyle and the desire to always have something to do fits quite well with pet ownership. Moreover, Järvikoski and Härkäpää (1987) also reported that their scale showed evidence of comprising more than one dimension. Thus, a multivariate analysis of the questionnaire data was carried out while comparing the 14 individual items of the questionnaire across the groups to explore the dimensionality of the differences that we had observed in the univariate analysis on the overall Type A scores.

A three-way multivariate analysis of variance (Pet Ownership Group × Age × Sex) was conducted with the 14 items in the Type A questionnaire as dependent variables. The results are complex, with a number of significant main effects and interactions. The multivariate main effect of group was significant (Wilks's lambda = 0.894; F (28, 966) = 2.00; $p = .002$), therefore, the dimensionality of this effect was explored (Chatfield & Collins, 1980). Tests on the residual roots showed that the solution was essentially unidimensional. The loadings (correlations) of each item on the canonical variable representing this dimension are presented in Table 11.1.

The items in Table 11.1 with the highest loadings are those that reflect a preference for being busy (with the exception of the item on being easily irritated). In contrast, the items with low loadings, indicating that they do not contribute to the dimension differentiating the pet ownership groups, include items on competitiveness, ambition, and possible hostility (interrupting). Thus, there is a reluctance to interpret these data as showing that the competitive and ambitious characteristics of classic Type A people are overrepresented in our sample of pet owners. The conclusion remains secure that the Type A personalities are not underrepresented among pet owners. This particular trait does not provide the basis for a noncausal explanation for the association between pet ownership and advantages for health.

In addition to participants' Type A scores, a number of other variables that could affect health outcomes were examined. These were tobacco and alcohol consumption, which are known to adversely affect health, and membership in clubs and societies, which could have beneficial effects through enhanced social networks, as in the indirect causal explanation outlined in the introduction. Ratings of self-perceived health and level of fitness were also analyzed.

No significant associations between any of these variables and pet ownership were found, with the exception of smoking behavior. A question asking participants whether they smoked did not differentiate pet owners from nonowners, but the number of cigarettes smoked per day was significantly greater among cat/dog owners than nonowners (Tukey's HSD, $p = .026$).

The survey also asked with whom the respondents shared their households. For analysis, we divided respondents into those who lived alone ($n = 59$); those whose households included one or more younger children, and possibly adults too ($n = 217$); and those who lived with other adults, such as older children or a spouse/partner, but no young children ($n = 235$). Thirty respondents did not supply answers to this section. This classification was then compared across the three pet-owning groups.

TABLE 11.1 Type A Scale Items and Their Loadings on the Dimension Underlying Differences Among the Pet Ownership Groups

Item	Role in scale: Type A people tendency to	Loading	Findings: Pet owners tendency to
I often do many things at once.	Agree	.608	Agree
I get impatient when I have to wait or queue.	Agree	.450	Agree
I am not easily irritated.	Disagree	.397	Disagree
I am very seldom in a hurry.	Disagree	.387	Disagree
I generally walk fast even if I am not in a hurry.	Agree	.380	Agree
I always try to be energetic and efficient.	Agree	.372	Agree
I often interrupt others when they are talking or finish their sentences for them.	Agree	.255	—
I am ambitious and always strive for new goals and better results.	Agree	.176	—
I enjoy life most when I have lots of work to do.	Agree	–.146	—
I do not like competing or setting difficult goals.	Disagree	.143	—
I do not usually compare my achievements with others.	Disagree	.126	—
I relax fully during my leisure time; work problems do not even cross my mind.	Disagree	–.097	—
I am always calm and easygoing.	Disagree	.091	—
I usually eat faster than other people.	Agree	.020	—

Pet ownership and type of pet owned was strongly associated with who, if anyone, composed the respondents' family households, χ^2 (4, $N = 511$) = 34.15, $p < .0005$. Respondents who had young children in their families were more likely to own pets of species other than cats or dogs (26.27%) than were respondents who lived with older children or just their partner (12.77%). Cat and dog ownership was similar for this group (40.55%) and for respondents who lived with older children or who lived with only a partner (42.98%). Respondents who lived alone were more likely not to own pets of any type (67.8%).

Discussion

The results of this study do not support the hypothesis that the presence of Type A behavior is associated with lower propensity to own a pet. Indeed, pet ownership was associated with higher Type A scores. Clearly, pet ownership is not underrepresented among Type A people. It should be emphasized, however, that pet ownership is most associated with high scores on those items of the Type A scale that focus on a desire for activity and energy. This is perhaps not surprising because owning a pet requires attention to its care, exercise, and well-being. Pet owners did not score more highly than nonowners on items relating to ambition, competitiveness, comparison of achievements with others, impatience with others, or inability to relax. This should not be interpreted that pet owners are less likely to exhibit these behaviors, merely that they display no difference on these items than nonowners. Thus, we conclude that the origin of the higher Type A scores displayed by pet owners is primarily due to their propensity for activity and keeping busy.

This raises an interesting question, which unfortunately cannot be addressed by this study, of whether there is a difference between high Type A scores that are primarily derived from scores on some items and high scores derived from other items. The study by Järvikoski and Härkäpää (1987) identified four factors in the 14-item scale. They labeled these as impatience, irritability, and speed (Factor 1); efficiency and activeness (Factor 2); competitiveness and aspiration (Factor 3); and tenseness and inability to relax (Factor 4). The study found that participants who experienced symptoms of severe angina pectoris had significantly higher overall Type A scores when compared with symptom-free participants and also had significantly higher scores on items loading on the factors of impatience and tenseness. The same distinction was also found for participants who experienced severe attacks of chest pain. Factors identified by Järvikoski and Härkäpää were not replicable in this study.

Whether it is overall behavior pattern or the presence of accompanying negative emotions that poses risk to health is not known. Brown (1986) points out that non-Type A persons may be as ambitious and have as much desire to achieve as Type A persons but that these desires serve to give them confidence and esteem, rather than to produce negative emotions such as goading or irritation. Similarly, Matthews (1987) reports in her meta-analysis that hostility and anxiety are significantly associated between Type A behavior and coronary heart disease.

The suggestion that the presence of negative emotions may be linked to adverse health outcomes can help identify other variables that could mediate a noncausal explanation for the association between pet ownership and health. Health psychology has long recognized the value of dispositional optimism (Scheier & Carver, 1987) and hardiness (Kobasa, 1979) as factors that influence positive health outcomes. As with our hypothesis that Type A persons may be underrepresented among pet owners, it is also plausible that people who are habitually pessimistic in their outlook may not desire to own pets. For example, focusing on the cost, responsibility, and potential problems that a pet might bring may discourage these people from acquiring pets. Similarly, people who are "nonhardy" in that they lack commitment, dislike challenge, or lack belief in their ability to control events may also choose not to own pets. Because both these factors are known to have positive effects on health outcome and could plausibly be related to propensity to own a pet, we recommend that these, and similar potential covariates of pet ownership, be investigated.

References

Anderson, W. P., Reid, C. M., & Jennings, G. L. (1992). Pet ownership and risk factors for cardiovascular disease. *Medical Journal of Australia, 157,* 298-301.

Brown, R. (1986). *Social psychology* (2nd ed.). New York: Free Press.

Chatfield, C., & Collins, A. J. (1980). *Introduction to multivariate analysis.* London: Chapman & Hall.

Friedman, M., & Rosenman, R. (1974). *Type A behavior and your heart.* New York: Knopf.

Friedmann, E., Katcher, A. H., Lynch, J. J., & Thomas, S. A. (1980). Animal companions and one year survival of patients after discharge from a coronary care unit. *Public Health Reports, 95,* 307-312.

Friedmann, E., Katcher, A. H., Thomas, S. A., Lynch, J. J., & Messent, P. R. (1983). Social interaction and blood pressure: Influence of animal companions. *Journal of Nervous and Mental Disease, 171*(8), 461-465.

Haynes, S. G., Feinleib, M., & Levine, S. (1978). The relationship of psychosocial factors to coronary heart disease in the Framingham Study II: Prevalence of coronary heart disease. *American Journal of Epidemiology, 107,* 384-402.

Järvikoski, A., & Härkäpää, K. (1987). A brief Type A scale and the occurrence of cardiovascular symptoms. *Scandinavian Journal of Rehabilitation Medicine, 19,* 115-120.

Kobasa, S. C. (1979). Stressful life events, personality and health: An inquiry into hardiness. *Journal of Personality and Social Psychology, 37,* 1-11.

Matthews, K. A. (1987). Coronary heart disease and Type A behaviors: Update on and alternative to the Booth-Kewley and Friedman (1987) quantitative review. *Psychological Bulletin, 104*(3), 373-380.

McNicholas, J., Collis, G. M., & Morley, I. E. (1995). Psychological support as a mechanism underlying health benefits associated with pet ownership. In S. M. Rutter, J. Rushen,

H. D. Randle, & J. C. Eddison (Eds.), *Proceedings of the 29th International Congress of the International Society for Applied Ethology* (pp. 119-121). Potters Bar, UK: Universities Federation for Animal Welfare.

McNicholas, J., Collis, G. M., Morley, I. E., & Lane, D. R. (1993). Social communication through a companion animal: The dog as a social catalyst. In M. Nichelmann, H. K. Wierenga, & S. Braun (Eds.), *Proceedings of the International Congress on Applied Ethology* (pp. 368-370). Berlin, Germany: Humboldt University.

Messent, P. R. (1983). Social facilitation of contact with other people by pet dogs. In A. H. Katcher & A. M. Beck (Eds.), *New perspectives in our lives with companion animals* (pp. 37-46). Philadelphia: University of Philadelphia Press.

Rime, B., Ucros, C. G., Bestgen, Y., & Jeanjean, M. (1989). Type A behavior pattern: Specific coronary risk factor or general disease-prone condition? *British Journal of Medical Psychology, 62,* 229-240.

Scheier, M. F., & Carver, C. S. (1987). Dispositional optimism and physical well-being: The influence of generalised outcome expectancies on health. *Journal of Personality, 55,* 169-210.

Serpell, J. A. (1991). Beneficial effects of pet ownership on some aspects of human health and behavior. *Journal of the Royal Society of Medicine, 84,* 717-720.

Pet Ownership, Social Support, and One-Year Survival After Acute Myocardial Infarction in the Cardiac Arrhythmia Suppression Trial (CAST) 12

Erika Friedmann
Sue A. Thomas

Abstract

Social support and pet ownership, a nonhuman form of social support, have both been associated with increased coronary artery disease survival. The independent effects of pet ownership, social support, disease severity, and other psychosocial factors on one-year survival after acute myocardial infarction are examined prospectively. The Cardiac Arrhythmia Suppression Trial provided physiologic data on a group of postmyocardial infarction patients with asymptomatic ventricular arrhythmias. An ancillary study provided psychosocial data, including pet ownership, social support, recent life events, future life events, anxiety, depression, coronary prone behavior, and expression of anger. Subjects ($N = 424$) were

AUTHORS' NOTE: This research was supported in part by grants from the Delta Society, NIH #5RO1 NR02043-01, and the PSC-CUNY Research Award Program. This chapter is reprinted by permission of the publisher from "Pet Ownership, Social Support, and One-Year Survival After Acute Myocardial Infarction in the Cardiac Arrhythmia Suppression Trial (CAST)" by Erika Friedmann and Sue A. Thomas, *American Journal of Cardiology*, Vol. 76, pp. 1213-1217. Copyright © 1995 by Excerpta Medica Inc.

randomly selected from patients attending participating Cardiac Arrhythmia Suppression Trial sites and completed baseline psychosocial questionnaires. One-year survival data were obtained from 369 (87%), of whom 112 (30.4%) owned pets and 20 (5.4%) died. Logistic regression indicates that high social support ($p <$ .068) and owning a pet ($p = $.085) tend to predict survival independent of physiologic severity, demographic, and other psychosocial factors. Dog owners ($n = 87$, 1 died) are significantly less likely to die within 1 year than persons who did not own dogs ($n = 282$, 19 died; $p < .05$); amount of social support is also an independent predictor of survival ($p = .065$). Both pet ownership and social support are significant predictors of survival, independent of the effects of the other psychosocial factors and physiologic status. These data confirm and extend previous findings relating pet ownership and social support to survival among patients with coronary artery disease.

Introduction

Support from nonhuman companions has been linked to coronary artery disease patient survival. Pet ownership was an independent predictor of 1-year survival in a prospective study of 92 patients admitted to a coronary care unit (Friedmann, Katcher, Lynch, & Thomas, 1980). The beneficial effects of pet ownership for survival were independent of marital status or living situation. The generalizability of the relation of pet ownership to survival of patients with coronary artery disease was limited by the small sample size, the nature of the sample, and measurement techniques. Recent research has documented that the presence of a pet is associated with decreased cardiovascular reactivity (Allen, Blascovich, Tomaka, & Kelsey, 1991; Friedmann, Katcher, Thomas, Lynch, & Messent, 1983) to stressors, that this stress-reducing effect is greater than the effect of the presence of a good friend (Allen et al., 1991), and that acquiring a pet leads to improved health status (Serpell, 1991). Furthermore, in a large epidemiological study, cardiovascular risk factors were greater among those who did not own than those who owned pets (Cardiac Arrhythmia Suppression Trial [CAST] Investigators, 1989). The current study further investigates the effect of pet ownership on 1-year survival among a well-defined group of postmyocardial infarction patients independent of the effects of physiologic, demographic, and other psychosocial variables.

Methods

Study

The current study was an independent project complementary to the Cardiac Arrhythmia Suppression Trial (CAST) and CAST II. These studies constituted a pharmacological test of the arrhythmia suppression and mortality hypothesis. Twelve of the 27 CAST clinical sites in the United States and 1 in Canada agreed to participate. The CAST began in 1987 with the randomization of subjects to 3 drugs, encainide, flecainide, or moricizine, or their matching placebos. When excess mortality was attributed to encainide and flecainide (April 19, 1989), randomization was halted (Anderson, Reid, & Jennings, 1992; Echt et al., 1991). The protocol was modified and permitted only the study of moricizine and its matching placebo, CAST II (Greene et al., 1992). The CAST II trial ended in September 1991 and concluded that patients with ventricular premature complexes after a myocardial infarction should not be routinely treated with anti-arrhythmic agents (Greene, Roden, Katz, Woosley, Salerno, & Henthorn, 1992).

Subject Recruitment

All patients who entered CAST or CAST II at each of the participating clinical sites during the period September 1987 to April 1993 were potentially eligible for recruitment into the study. When the baseline information was transmitted to the CAST coordinating center, the center randomly assigned subjects to be approached to participate in the study. Additional informed consent was required for participation; 12% declined to participate.

Procedure

Subjects were asked to participate in this study while they were at the CAST clinical site. CAST clinical trial personnel recruited the participants and administered all forms. At baseline, each subject completed the following indices: social support questionnaire-6 (SSQ6; Sarason, Sarason, Sheann, & Pierce, 1987), social readjustment rating scale (Holmes & Rahe, 1967), pet ownership/attachment survey, state-trait anxiety inventory (Spielberger, Lushene, & Gorsuch, 1972), self-rating depression scale (Zung, 1965), Jenkins activity survey (Jenkins, Zyzanski, & Rosenman, 1979), and expression of anger scale (Spielberger, Johnson, Russel, Crane, Jacobs, & Worden, 1985). In addition, physiologic data including left ventricular ejection fraction, presence of myocardial ischemia, congestive heart failure, New York Heart Association and Canadian Cardiovascular classifications, number of prior myocardial infarctions, presence of diabetes mellitus, and family medical history were obtained from the CAST coordinating center data bank.

Mortality data were obtained by CAST clinical site personnel from physicians, family members, and medical records. One-year survivors were participants who were alive 1 year after baseline; non-survivors were those whose date of death was less than 1 year after baseline.

Instruments

The SSQ6 was used to quantify both the amount of and satisfaction with social support perceived by a patient. The SSQ6 provides a list of six circumstances potentially requiring social support and asks the respondent who they could rely on for help in each situation (amount) and how satisfied they would be with the help they received in each situation (satisfaction; Sarason, Levine, Basham, & Sarason, 1983; Sarason, Sarason, & Sheann, 1986; Sarason et al., 1987). Persons who owned one or more dogs were classified as dog owners, and those who owned one or more cats were classified as cat owners.

Pet ownership status was assessed with 1 item contained in a 10-item pet demographic questionnaire. The participant was asked to list the number and type of pets in the home and provide information on pet restrictions in the residence. The question "Do any of the above pets belong to you?" was used to classify persons as pet owners.

Several psychosocial factors were also assessed at baseline: state and trait anxiety, depression, anger expressed inward and outward, coronary prone behavior, and stressful life events occurring in the recent past and expected to occur in the near future.

Subjects

A total of 424 subjects were recruited into the study. One-year survival status was obtained from 369 (87%) of the participants. Of the 55 participants lost to follow-up, 54 (98%) had been followed for < 1 year when CAST II ended prematurely. A characterization of the subjects according to demographic and physiologic characteristics is included in Table 12.1

One hundred and twelve (30.4%) participants owned pets. This is somewhat lower than reports that 41% of retired couples own pets and that

Variable	n (%)	Mean +/–SD
TABLE 12.1 Characterization of 369 Participants According to Baseline Demographic and Physiological Variables		
Male	314	(85.1%)
White	280	(75.9%)
Black	57	(15.4%)
Married	266	(72.1%)
CAST active treatment	43	(11.7%)
Congestive heart failure	52	(14.2%)
Diabetes mellitus	67	(18.9%)
Education		
< High school	89	(24.2%)
High school graduate	108	(29.3%)
>/= College graduate	62	(16.8%)
Retired	205	(55.6%)
Employed full-time	84	(22.8%)
Age (years)	62.83	+/– 9.17
Survival length (years)	1.62	+/– 0.59
Ejection fraction (%)	38.19	+/– 9.63
Previous myocardial infarctions	144	(39.0%)
Runs of ventricular tachycardia	86	(23.3%)

NOTE: Values are expressed as number (%) or as mean +/– *SD*. CAST = Cardiac Arrhythmia Suppression Trial.

the proportion of couples owning pets increases as the ages of the couples decreases (Rowan, 1992). The pet owners consisted of 87 persons who kept at least 1 dog and 44 who kept at least 1 cat; 24 of these pet owners kept both cats and dogs. Other pets included birds, fish, ducks, horses, snakes, and rabbits.

Potential differences in baseline psychosocial and physiologic status between those who completed follow-up and those who did not were examined. The physiologic profile included ejection fraction, diabetes mellitus, runs of ventricular arrhythmias, medication group (active or nonactive), sex, and age. All psychosocial variables assessed at baseline were included in the psychosocial profile of participants. Neither the physiologic (Wilks's lambda = .9808, F [6, 416] = 1.36, p = .231) nor the psychosocial (Wilks's lambda = .9652, F [10, 396] = 1.43, p = .165) profiles of the 2 groups differed significantly.

Statistical analysis

Chi-square analyses were used to examine the univariate relation between pet ownership and survival status. The possibility that pet ownership made a significant independent contribution to survival while controlling for physiologic severity of the illness was examined. Logistic regression with the physiologic severity and demographic variables (age, diabetes mellitus, left ventricular ejection fraction, runs of ventricular premature depolarization, and sex), the psychosocial variables and pet ownership were entered simultaneously to evaluate the independent contributions of each variable. Similar logistic regression analyses were performed to assess the effect of dog and cat ownership both individually and in combination on survival status. A stepwise hierarchical logistic regression was used to examine the effects of the physiologic variables (step 1), social support amount (step 2), and cat ownership (step 3) on survival. Differences in physiologic status between those who own dogs and those who do not and those who do and do not survive were examined with a 2-way multivariate analysis of variance. Multivariate analyses of variance were used to examine differences in physiologic and psychosocial status between dog and cat owners.

Results

Twenty of the 369 participants (5.4%) in the study died within 1 year. When the frequency of deaths among pet owners and non-owners was compared, there was no significant relation between pet ownership and 1-year survival (see Table 12.2). The frequencies of dog and cat ownership were sufficient to examine each separately in relation to survival status. There was a significant univariate relation between dog ownership and survival (χ^2 [1 *df*, $N = 369$] $= 4.05, p = .044$; see Table 12.2) but not between cat ownership and survival. Dog owners were more likely to be alive 1 year after the baseline assessment than people who did not own dogs.

Pet Ownership and Survival

The combination of the physiologic and psychosocial variables and pet ownership was 95.74% accurate at predicting membership in the correct survival group, 99% accurate for survivors, and 37% accurate for non-

TABLE 12.2   One-Year Survival Status According to Pet Ownership, Dog Ownership, and Cat Ownership

Ownership Status	Survived (Number of Subjects)	Died (Number of Subjects)	Chi-Square
No pets	246	16	
Pets	103	4	1.07
No dogs	263	19	
Dogs	86	1	4.05*
No cats	308	17	
Cats	41	3	.19

$p < .05$

survivors (χ^2 [1 df, $n = 71$] = 77.44, $p < .0001$). As expected, physiologic variables (ejection fraction, diabetes mellitus, and runs of ventricular premature beats) were significant, independent predictors of survival. Pet ownership tended to be independently related to survival ($p = .085$). In the logistic regression analysis, when the effects of the physiologic and other psychosocial variables were controlled, pet owners tended to be more likely to survive 1 year than non-owners.

The specific psychosocial variables that contributed to prediction of survival were then examined. The amount of social support also made a significant independent contribution to survival. Participants with greater amounts of social support were more likely to survive 1 year, controlling for the effects of all other psychosocial and physiologic variables. Two additional psychosocial variables tended to make independent contributions to survival status: lower state anxiety ($p = .087$), and greater expectations of future life changes ($p = .065$).

Dog Owners, Cat Owners, and Survival

Physiologic and psychosocial variables and cat and dog ownership were entered into a logistic regression equation to predict 1-year survival status. Survival status was predicted well; 17.5% of the variance in survival was explained (model χ^2 [$df = 18$, $n = 352$] = 75.93, $p < .0001$; goodness of fit [$df = 333$] = 103.42, $p = 1.00$). The combination of these variables predicted survival status correctly 95.7% of the time. Survival status was predicted correctly for 98.8% of those who actually survived 1 year and for 42.1% of those who actually died within 1 year. As would be expected, physiologic variables were the best independent predictors of survival: ejection fraction ($R = -.2352, p = .0007$, Exp[B] = .8688), runs ($R = -.2211, p = .0012$, Exp[B] = .1167), and diabetes mellitus ($R = -.1652, p = .014$, Exp[B] = .1658). Dog ownership made a significant independent contribution to survival status ($R = .1204, p = .02$, Exp[B] = .0687). Social support also tended to be related to survival status ($R = .0628, p = .05$, Exp[B] = .9355). Increased likelihood of 1-year survival was associated with higher ejection fractions, not having diabetes mellitus, not having runs of ventricular premature beats, not owning a cat, owning a dog, and having greater amounts of social support. Thus, dog ownership made a significant positive contribution to survival status, while controlling for cat ownership, physiologic status, and the other psychosocial factors, including social support.

Dog Owners and Survival

Physiologic and psychosocial variables and dog ownership were entered into a logistic regression equation to predict 1-year survival status. Survival status was predicted well; 24% of the variance in survival was explained (model χ^2 [$df = 17, n = 352$] = 70.84 , $p < .0001$; goodness of fit [$df = 334$] = 156.28 $p = 1.0$). The combination of these variables predicted survival status correctly 96% of the time. Survival status was predicted correctly for 99.1% of those who actually survived 1 year and for 42.1% of those who actually died within 1 year. As would be expected, physiologic variables were the best independent predictors of survival: ejection fraction ($R = -.2538, p = .0004$, Exp[B] = .8697), runs ($R = -.2253, p = .001$, Exp[B] =.1243), and diabetes mellitus ($R = -.1496, p = .01$, Exp[B] = .1957). Among the psychosocial variables dog ownership ($R = .0720, p = .05$, Exp[B] = .1068) and the amount of social support ($R = .0508, p = .05$, Exp[B] = .9420) made significant independent contributions to survival status. Increased likelihood of 1-year survival was associated with higher ejection fractions, not having diabetes mellitus, not having runs of ventricular premature beats, owning a dog, and having greater amounts of social support. Thus, dog ownership made a contribution to survival status, while controlling for both physiologic status and the other psychosocial factors, including social support.

Health Status, Dog Owners, and Survival

Researchers have previously suggested that any differences in health status between pet owners and non-owners could be a result of healthier people choosing to own pets, particularly dogs. The current study afforded the opportunity to examine this explanation directly among a group of patients with coronary artery disease. The physiologic profiles of those who do and do not own dogs and those who do and do not survive were compared. There is no evidence that differences in the physiologic status of dog owners and non-owners are responsible for the differences in 1-year survival between those who do and do not own dogs (Wilks's lambda = .977, F [6, 359] = 1.41, p = .21). The physiologic profile of those who owned dogs did not differ significantly from that of those who did not (Wilks's lambda = .985, F [6, 359] = 0.94, p = .47; see Figure 12.1). As would be expected, the physiologic profile of those who survived was significantly different from the profile of those who did not (Wilks's lambda = .925, F [6, 359] = 4.84, p < .001; see Figure 12.2).

Cat Owners and Survival

Physiologic and psychosocial variables and cat ownership were entered into a logistic regression equation to predict 1-year survival status. Survival status was predicted well; 25.6% of the variance in survival was explained (model χ^2 [df = 17, n = 352] = 69.77, p < .0001; goodness of fit [df = 334] = 136.29, p = 1.00). The combination of these variables predicted survival status correctly 96% of the time. Survival status was predicted correctly for 99.1% of those who actually survived 1 year and for 42.1% of those who actually died within 1 year. Increased likelihood of survival was associated with higher ejection fraction, not having diabetes mellitus, not having runs of ventricular premature beats, being a man (R = .1516, p = .02, Exp[B] = 5.76) and not owning a cat (R = .1601, p = .03, Exp[B] = 8.01). Cat ownership contributed to survival contrary to the hypothesized direction.

Cat Owners, Social Support, and Survival

The interrelation of social support, cat ownership, and survival was examined more closely. When the independent effect of social support was

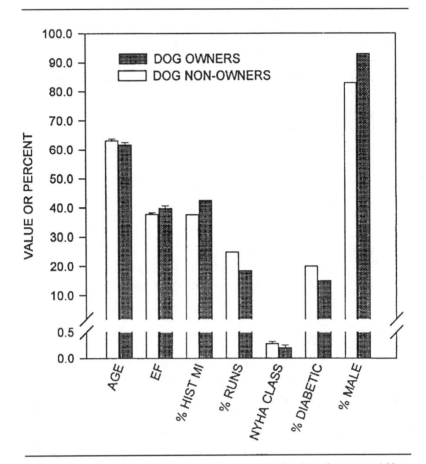

Figure 12.1. Comparison of Physiological Profiles for Dog Owners and Non-Owners

NOTES: Comparison of baseline physiologic profiles of participants who owned ($n = 87$) and did not own dogs ($n = 272$). Age is expressed in years; EF = percentage left ventricular ejection fraction; HIST MI = history of at least one myocardial infarction before the CAST qualifying myocardial infarction; NYHA = New York Heart Association congestive heart failure classification; RUNS = having runs of ventricular tachycardia on 24-hour Holter monitor.

entered before cat ownership, cat ownership did not make a significant contribution to survival. Thus the relation of cat ownership to survival was not independent of social support.

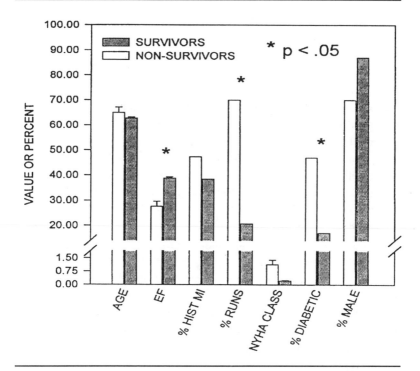

Figure 12.2. Comparison of Physiological Profiles for One-Year Survivors and Non-Survivors

NOTES: Comparison of baseline physiologic profiles according to survival status; the 349 participants who were alive 1 year after baseline (survivors) were compared with the 20 participants who did within 1 year of baseline (non-survivors). Age is expressed in years. Abbreviations as in Figure 12.1.

Dog Owners, Cat Owners, and Physiologic Status

Physiologic profiles of participants who owned only cats and participants who owned dogs were compared. The physiologic profiles of the 87 persons who owned dogs did differ from the profiles of the 20 who owned only cats (F [6, 115] = 2.61, p = .012). The difference was largely in the sex of the subjects, 11.4% of the cat owners were women compared with 6.9% of the dog owners. The psychosocial profiles of the dog and cat owners did not differ (F [10, 108] = .92, p = .514).

Discussion

In this study of 369 participants in CAST, who were followed for at least 1 year, dog ownership and social support made significant independent contributions to survival beyond the effects of the physiologic measures of the severity of the cardiovascular disease. These positive findings support and increase the generalizability of the previous finding that pet ownership was related to survival of patients with coronary artery disease, independent of social support (Friedmann et al., 1980). Dog ownership and amount of social support were independent predictors of survival. Although owning a dog had a positive influence on health, that effect was complementary to, rather than a substitute for, other sources of social support. In contrast, cat ownership was not related to survival and was not independent of social support.

On the basis of the current study, one should not conclude that cat ownership is harmful. It is likely that differences in other characteristics are responsible both for cat ownership and the apparent lower survival of cat owners. In a recent study (Serpell, 1991), cat owners were significantly more likely to be sedentary than people who owned dogs and those who did not own any pets. Although the current study did not include assessment of exercise habits, it is possible that sedentary persons were less likely to survive.

Investigation of the relation of cat ownership to other factors which might also be related to survival was possible. None of the women who owned cats also owned dogs, whereas 24 of the 39 men who owned cats also owned dogs. Examination of differences between cat and dog owners revealed that whereas the psychosocial profiles of the 2 groups did not differ, the physiologic profiles did. A much higher percentage of cat (11.4%) than of dog owners (6.9%) were women. Overall, women had higher 1-year mortality ($p < .01$, hazard ration = 1.9) than men in CAST (Gorkin et al., 1994). Because only 5 women owned cats, further study is necessary to quantify the interrelation between survival, social support, and cat ownership.

Attachment to a pet may be responsible for differences in cardiovascular benefits of pets among pet owners (Friedmann, 1995). In the current study, pet ownership was defined as claiming a pet as one's own rather than just having a pet in the household. Whereas those who own both dogs and cats have been reported to have less attachment to their cats than their dogs, this difference does not appear to be responsible for the observed differences in mortality between dog and cat owners. In the current study, among men who owned only cats, the mortality rate was significantly higher (2 of 15) than among those who owned dogs with or without cats (0 of 81). There were not large differences in mortality among women (1 of 5, 1 of 6, respectively).

In the current study, social support was the only psychosocial variable, in addition to dog ownership, that was an independent predictor of survival. Patients with greater amounts of social support, as measured on the 6-item SSQ-6 scale, were more likely to survive than those with lesser amounts. This finding is consistent with the multivariate findings for the 647 participants in the CAST placebo group (Gorkin et al., 1994) in which social support, as measured with 1 item, was the only baseline psychosocial variable that was related to survival in multivariate analysis. It was also consistent with the findings for the 194 men and women in the Established Populations for the Epidemiologic Study of the Elderly Population who were hospitalized with myocardial infarctions in 2 New Haven hospitals (Berkman, Leo-Summers, & Horwitz, 1992). In that study, the number of persons available to provide support, but not integration into social networks, was related to survival. In these studies, the type of social support that was related to survival was a measure of the availability of other persons to provide support when needed. This contrasts with other types of social support that include satisfaction with social support (the current study; Williams et al., 1992), the amount of support patients thought they actually needed, and integration into social networks (Berkman et al., 1992), which were not related to survival of patients with coronary artery disease.

The powerful detrimental drug effects in CAST made it a difficult vehicle for evaluating the impact of psychosocial factors on survival (Gorkin et al., 1994). This problem was minimized in the current study because a majority of patients (88.3%) were not taking active medication. Furthermore, there were no significant differences in the distribution of active medication between pet owners (12.5%) and non-owners (10.9%).

Pets are theorized to act as buffers to stress. Pet ownership is proposed to afford several benefits to their owners, including decreases in anxiety (Wilson, 1991) and sympathetic nervous system arousal (Friedmann, 1995; Friedmann et al., 1983) in response to stressors. In addition, people who acquire pets report improved health over the subsequent months compared with controls (Serpell, 1991), and pet owners receiving Medicaid make fewer visits to their physicians than non-owners (Siegel, 1990). These studies concur with the current study in supporting better health status or outcome among pet owners than among non-owners.

It has been suggested that dog owners might be healthier than owners of other pets and thus the better survival among dog owners is a reflection of their better physiologic status. The basis for conjecture is that caring for a dog often requires more work than needed to keep other pets. Accordingly, one would expect differences in physiologic status between dog owners and those who did not own dogs to account for the increased likelihood of survival among dog owners. This conjecture was not supported in the current study. There were no differences in physiologic status between those who own dogs and either all subjects or owners of other pets.

Furthermore, the contributions of pet and dog ownership to survival were independent of the contributions of the physiologic factors that predict survival.

The current study provides strong evidence that pet ownership, and dog ownership in particular, promotes cardiovascular health independent of social support and the physiologic severity of the illness. Additional research with larger samples is needed to investigate the interrelations between cat ownership, social support, and cardiovascular health.

References

Allen, K. M., Blascovich, J., Tomaka, J., Kelsey, R. M. (1991). Presence of human friends and pet dogs as moderators of autonomic responses to stress in women. *Journal of Personality and Social Psychology, 61*, 582-589.

Anderson, W., Reid, P., & Jennings, G. L.. (1992). Pet ownership and risk factors for cardiovascular disease. *Medical Journal of Australia, 157*, 298-301.

Berkman, L. F., Leo-Summers, L., & Horwitz, R. I. (1992). Emotional support and survival after myocardial infarction. *Annals of Internal Medicine, 117*, 1003-1009.

Cardiac Arrhythmia Suppression Trial (CAST) Investigators. (1989). Preliminary report: Effect of encainide and flecainide on mortality in a randomized trial of arrhythmia suppression after myocardial infarction. *New England Journal of Medicine, 321*, 406-412.

Echt, D. S., Liebson, P. R., Mitchell, L. B., Peters, R. W., Obias-Manno, D., Barker, A. H., Arensberg, D., Baker, A., Friedman, L., Greene, H. L., Hunter, M. L., Richardson, D. W. (1991). Mortality and morbidity in patients receiving encainide, flecainide, or placebo: The Cardiac Arrhythmia Suppression Trial. *New England Journal of Medicine, 324*, 781-788.

Friedmann, E. (1995). The role of pets in enhancing human well-being: Physiological effects. In I. Robinson (Ed.), *Waltham book of human-animal interactions*. Oxford, UK: Pergamon.

Friedmann, E., Katcher, A. H., Lynch, J. J., & Thomas, S. A. (1980). Animal companions and one year survival of patients after discharge from a coronary care unit. *Public Health Reports, 95,* 307-312.

Friedmann, E., Katcher, A. H., Thomas, S. A., Lynch, J. J., & Messent, P. R. (1983). Social interaction and blood pressure: The influence of animal companions. *Journal of Nervous and Mental Disease, 171,* 461-465.

Gorkin, L., Schron, E. B., Brooks, M. M., Wiklund, I., Kellen, J., Verter, J., Schoenberger, J. A., Pawitan, Y., Morris, M., & Shumaker, S. (1994). Psychosocial predictors of mortality in the Cardiac Arrhythmia Suppression Trial (CAST-1). *American Journal of Cardiology, 21,* 263-267.

Greene, H. L., Roden, D. M., Katz, R. J., Woosley, R. L., Salerno, D. M., & Henthorn, R. W. (1992). The Cardiac Arrhythmia Suppression Trial: First CAST . . . then CAST-II. *American Journal of Cardiology, 19,* 894-898.

Holmes, T. H., & Rahe, R. H. (1967). The social readjustment rating scale. *Journal of Psychosomatic Research, 11,* 213-218.

Jenkins, C. D., Zyzanski, S. J., & Rosenman, R. H. (1979). *Jenkins activity survey manual.* New York: Psychological Corporation.

Rowan, A. (1992). Companion animal demographics and unwanted animals in the United States. *Anthrozoös, 5,* 222-225.

Sarason, I. G., Levine, H. M., Basham, R. B., Sarason, B. R. (1983). Assessing social support: The social support questionnaire. *Journal of Personality and Social Psychology, 44,* 127-139.

Sarason, I. G., Sarason, B. R., & Sheann, E. N. (1986). Social support as an individual difference variable: Its stability, origins, and relational aspects. *Journal of Personality and Social Psychology, 50,* 845-855.

Sarason, I. G., Sarason, B. R., Sheann, E. N., & Pierce, G. (1987). A brief measure of social support: Practical and theoretical implications. *Journal of Social and Personal Relationships, 4,* 497-510.

Serpell, J. A. (1991). Beneficial effects of pet ownership on some aspects of human health. *Journal of the Royal Society of Medicine, 84,* 717-720.

Siegel, J. M. (1990). Stressful life events and use of physician services among the elderly: The moderating role of pet ownership. *Journal of Personality and Social Psychology, 58,* 1081-1086.

Spielberger, C. D., Johnson, E. H., Russell, S. F., Crane, R. J., Jacobs, J. A., & Worden, T. J. (1985). The experience and expression of anger: Construction and validation of anger expression scale. In M. A. Chesney & R. H. Rosenman (Eds.), *Anger and hostility in cardiovascular and behavioral disorders* (pp. 5-30). New York: Hemisphere/McGraw-Hill.

Spielberger, C. D., Lushene, R. E., & Gorsuch, R. L. (1972). *STAI manual.* Palo Alto, CA: Consulting Psychologist Press.

Williams, R. B., Barefoot, J. C., Califf, R. M., Haney, T. L., Saunders, W. B., Pryor, D. B., Hlatky, M. A., Siegler, I. C., & Mark, D. B. (1992). Prognostic importance of social and economic resources among medically treated patients with angiographically documented coronary artery disease. *Journal of the American Medical Association, 267,* 520-525.

Wilson, C. C. (1991). The pet as an anxiolytic intervention. *Journal of Nervous and Mental Disease, 179,* 482-489.

Zung, W. K. (1965). A self-rating depression scale. *Archives of General Psychiatry, 12,* 63-70.

The Effect of a Therapy Dog on Socialization and Physiological Indicators of Stress in Persons Diagnosed With Alzheimer's Disease **13**

Kathryn Batson
Barbara McCabe
Mara M. Baun
Carol Wilson

Abstract

This study examined the effect of the presence of a therapy dog on socialization and physiological indicators of stress in individuals diagnosed with Alzheimer's disease. A within-participants, repeated measures experimental design was used to measure heart rate, blood pressure (Kendall Model 8200 blood pressure monitor, Kendall™ Company Hospital Products, Boston, MA), and skin temperature (YSI Tele-Thermometer, Yellow Springs Instrument Company, Inc., Yellow Springs, OH) every 2 minutes during 10-minute sessions with or without a dog present. Sessions were videotaped for later coding (Daubenmire, White, Heinzerling, Ashton, & Searles, 1977). Frequency scores for smiles ($t = 2.33, p < .05$), tactile contact ($t = 4.35, p < .01$), looks ($t = 2.78, p < .05$), physical

AUTHORS' NOTE: Please send correspondence to Mara M. Baun, D.N.Sc., F.A.A.N., University of Nebraska Medical Center, College of Nursing, 600 S. 42nd Street, Omaha, NE 69198-5330.

warmth ($t = 4.35, p < .01$), and praise $t = 2.79, p < .01$) and duration scores for smiles ($t = 3.30, p < .01$), tactile contact ($t = 2.83, p < .01$), looks ($t = 4.42, p < .01$), and leans toward ($t = 2.08, p < .05$) were significantly higher when the pet was present, but the physiological indicators were not. Findings suggest that pets can serve as a useful intervention for increasing socialization for persons with Alzheimer's disease.

Alzheimer's disease (AD) is recognized as the fifth leading cause of disability and the fourth leading cause of death in the United States (U.S. Congress, 1987). A progressive brain disorder, Alzheimer's disease is characterized by impairments in a wide spectrum of cognitive abilities including memory, language, judgment, and abstract reasoning (American Psychiatric Association, 1987). Individuals with AD may live from 7 to 20 years postdiagnosis of AD (Katzman & Jackson, 1991) and constitute a large portion of the nursing home population (Brody, Lawton, & Liebowitz, 1984). It is important to identify interventions that increase the quality of life of persons with AD and that may compensate for the deterioration in functioning.

The global deterioration that occurs in persons with AD results in numerous difficulties for the AD individual and the caregiver. Communication problems have been identified as the sixth most common problem faced by AD caregivers. As the individual's language ability becomes increasingly impaired, communication difficulties increase (Lee, 1991). The resulting disturbed communication patterns that occur with AD have a profound effect on quality of life. As the disease progresses, it appears that the amount of time the person with AD spends interacting with others decreases (Kongable, Stolley, & Buckwalter, 1990). Because communication is a basic human need that serves to maintain the individual's contact with the environment while promoting a sense of security, efforts must be made to identify alternative approaches that enhance communication efforts for the person with AD.

Cognitive impairment that accompanies AD causes difficulty in understanding incoming information, resulting in symptoms of agitation and stress that often culminate in a catastrophic reaction (Lee, 1991). Communication and stress are interactive in that lowered stress is related to an increased ability to communicate, and increased communication ability is associated with decreased stress (Hall & Buckwalter, 1987; Mace & Rabins, 1991). The majority of persons with AD are admitted to long-term care facilities just as they have lost many of their communication skills. The stress of institutionalization, plus the stress of decreased communication abilities, places these persons at high risk for many untoward reactions (Lee, 1991). Hall and Buckwalter have demonstrated the calming effect of matching environmental stimuli and environmental demands to the level of cognitive functioning of the person with AD.

Within the last decade, there has been an increasing interest in the therapeutic effects of companion animals on human beings. Short-term interactions with companion animals have resulted in significantly increased interactive behaviors among both mentally sound (Buelt, Bergstrom, Baun, & Langston, 1985) and mentally impaired (Brunmeier, McArthur, Baun, & Bergstrom, 1986) institutionalized older persons. Although in the latter study, none of the participants had diagnoses of AD, a similar study of patients with AD residing in a special care unit showed increased communicative behaviors in the presence of a dog (Kongable, Buckwalter, & Stolley, 1989).

Long-term association of companion animals with persons with Alzheimer's living in the home has been associated with fewer episodes of verbal aggression and anxiety compared with those not exposed to companion animals (Fritz, Farver, Kass, & Hart, 1995). Persons with Alzheimer's who were attached to their pets also had fewer reported mood disorders. When the effects of companion animals on the caregivers of persons with Alzheimer's were studied, few benefits were identified (Fritz, Farver, Hart, & Kass, 1996).

Short-term interactions with companion animals have resulted in physiologic effects indicative of relaxation (e.g., blood pressure, heart rate, and peripheral skin temperature (Baun, Bergstrom, Langston, & Thoma, 1984; Grossberg & Alf, 1985; Schuelke et al., 1991-1992). These effects on the cardiovascular and neural-endocrine systems may be mechanisms by which interaction with companion animals produces its calming effects. If these physiologic effects could be demonstrated also in persons with Alzheimer's disease under controlled conditions, findings could support future study of the introduction of a companion animal into the less well controlled general living areas of institutionalized persons with Alzheimer's. Thus, the purposes of this study were to examine the effect of the short-term presence of a therapy dog on socialization and physiological indicators of stress for those with AD and to determine if changes in socialization when the therapy dog was present were related to level of dementia.

Method

Setting and Sample

Twenty-five participants were recruited for the study. Data from only 22 participants were usable for the analysis of socialization variables, and data from only 21 participants could be used for analysis of the physiological variables. Three long-term care facilities located either in midsized midwestern cities or in a small midwestern town were the study sites. The facilities chosen contained special care units designed to meet the needs of residents with dementia. Inclusion criteria for participants were diagnosis of probable AD, the ability to sit in a chair or wheelchair for at least 20 minutes, consent from the legally authorized representative of the participant for participation in the study, and assent by the participant. Individuals who had known allergies to dogs; had a history of negative reactions to dogs; or had more than a moderate impairment of vision, touch, or hearing were excluded.

Approval for this study was obtained from the Institutional Review Board for the Protection of Human Subjects and from the Institutional Animal Care and Use Committee of the University of Nebraska Medical Center. Each facility also gave permission to conduct the study at its respective institution. Because of the dependent status of the participants, informed consent was obtained from their legally authorized representatives, and verbal assent was obtained from the participants themselves. The head nurse on each special care unit identified residents meeting the study criteria. The potential participant's legally authorized representative was given a standard letter describing the research project and asking for permission to be contacted by the investigator. If permission was given, the investigator contacted the legally authorized representative and made an appointment to explain the purposes and methods of the study. Following the explanation, if permission to include the participant in the study was granted, the legally authorized representative signed the consent form and was given a copy of the form. Prior to escorting the participant to the session, the investigator read a letter of assent to the participant and did not proceed with the study if the participant actively dissented.

Design

A within-participants, repeated measures experimental design was used with the therapy dog as the independent variable. The dog was a trained miniature schnauzer certified as a therapy dog. Dependent variables were the social interaction variables of verbalizations, looks, smile, leans toward stimulus, tactile contact, praise, physical warmth, temporal response time and the physiological variables of heart rate, systolic and diastolic blood pressure, mean arterial pressure, and skin temperature. The Burke Dementia Scale was used to assess each participant's severity of impairment because of AD. Demographic data included gender, age, years diagnosed with AD, months on special care unit, other medical diagnoses, and currently prescribed medication.

Instruments

Social Interaction

Social interaction variables have been used in previous research with older participants and were derived from coding protocols by Daubenmire, White, Heinzerling, Ashton, and Searles (1977) and Kogan and Gordon (1975). Verbalizations, looks, smiles, tactile contact, and leans toward were coded by frequency and duration; physical warmth and praise were coded by frequency only; temporal response time was measured by duration only. Duration was the total number of seconds the behavior occurred. To determine frequency, the 10-minute session was subdivided into 15 segments. The total score represented the number of segments in which the behavior occurred. As suggested by Kongable et al. (1989), sessions were videotaped. The videotape allowed variables to be coded more than one time to improve accuracy. To increase reliability, all variables were coded at least two times on different days. Because it was not possible to be blinded to the experimental or control conditions, the tapes were coded on different days without reference to the score from the other condition. If duration measures differed by more than 10 seconds or if frequency scores differed by greater than one occurrence, the tape was coded a third time, and the average of the two closest measures was used.

Blood Pressure and Heart Rate

Blood pressure and heart rate were measured with the Kendall Model 8200 blood pressure monitor (Kendall™ Company Hospital Products, Boston, MA). The device is automatic and was set to make measurements at 2-minute intervals. The blood pressure monitor was calibrated by a biomedical instrumentation research laboratory prior to the study. The monitor contains a microcomputer that automatically calibrates a pressure transducer zero reference before each measurement. Blood pressure data were measured in millimeters of mercury (mmHg), and heart rate data were recorded in beats per minute. Mean arterial pressure was calculated using the following formula: mean arterial pressure = diastolic pressure + ⅓ (systolic pressure – diastolic pressure) (Bern & Levy, 1983).

Peripheral Skin Temperature

Peripheral skin temperature was measured in Fahrenheit and recorded every 2 minutes using a YSI Tele-Thermometer (Yellow Springs Instrument Company, Inc., Yellow Springs, OH). The thermometer was calibrated by a biomedical instrumentation research laboratory immediately prior to the study by comparing the thermistor probe to a National Bureau of Standards-calibrated Fahrenheit mercury thermometer.

Dementia

Severity of dementia was rated using the Burke Dementia Scale (Haycox, 1984). Theoretical range of scores is 0 (*no deficit*) to 48 (*deficit*). The scale correlates well with clinical impressions of dementia, $r = .90$.

Procedure

Patients participated in 10-minute sessions on 2 different days: 1 day with and 1 day without the dog present. A tale of random numbers was used to assign the order of conditions. Two investigators were present during all sessions; one to interact with the resident and one to record physiological data. The same investigator always interacted with the participants. Identical procedures and personnel were used in all sites. All sessions were conducted between 8:30 a.m. and 1:30 p.m.

Each participant was escorted to a private room on the special care unit. The procedure was explained, and the equipment was placed on the

TABLE 13.1   Socialization Variables

Variables	Frequency (Number of Segments)	Duration (Seconds)
Leans toward		
Experimental	0.3	0.7*
Control	0.5	0.09
Smiles		
Experimental	5.6*	39.1**
Control	3.8	15.6
Tactile Contact		
Experimental	5.1**	100.5**
Control	0	0
Looks		
Experimental	12.4*	244.2**
Control	9.2	97.5
Verbalization		
Experimental	12.7	145.5
Control	12.7	97.5
Praise		
Experimental	1.7**	
Control	0.2	
Physical Warmth		
Experimental	4.7**	
Control	0	
Temporal Response		
Experimental		0.01
Control		0.01

*$p < .05$; **$p < .01$.

participant. The blood pressure cuff was attached to the left arm, and the skin temperature probe was taped to the left forefinger to allow the right arm to be free to pet the dog.

Four minutes of baseline physiological data were recorded, followed by a standardized introduction to either the investigator or the investigator and the therapy dog. After the introduction, a conversation script consisting of open-ended questions suitable for individuals diagnosed with AD was used by the investigator if verbalization was not initiated by the participant. The physiological variables were measured every 2 minutes during both sessions. To prevent effects on skin temperature from blood pressure cuff inflation, skin temperature was recorded immediately prior to the inflation of the blood pressure cuff.

Data Analysis

Socialization data were analyzed using dependent *t*-tests. Repeated measures analysis of variance (ANOVA) were used for physiological data. Pearson product moment correlations and split-plot ANOVA were used to determine the relationship between the level of dementia and socialization variables. Demographics were analyzed using descriptive statistics.

Results

The sample included 12 women and 10 men with a mean age of 77.9 (range = 62 to 96) years. Participants had resided on the special care unit an average of 10.1 (range = 2 to 29) months, had been diagnosed with AD for a mean of 3.9 (range = 1 to 11) years, and had a mean Burke Dementia Scale score of 21.8 (range = 4 - 34).

Dependent *t*-tests revealed significant differences when the dog was present for the following socialization variables: frequency scores for smiles ($t = 2.33$, $p < .05$), tactile contact ($t = 4.35$, $p < .01$), looks ($t = 2.78$, $p < .05$), physical warmth ($t = 4.35$, $p < .01$), and praise ($t = 2.79$, $p < .01$) and duration of leans toward ($t = 2.08$, $p < .05$), smiles ($t = 3.30$, $p < .01$), tactile contact ($t = 2.83$, $p < .01$), and looks ($t = 4.42$, $p < .01$). See Table 13.1.

As shown in Table 13.2, Pearson product moment correlation coefficients indicated significant relationships between Burke Dementia Scale rating and a number of socialization variables when the dog was present: frequency of smiles, physical warmth, and praise and duration of looks and verbalization. To determine whether severity of dementia affected interactions with the investigator alone in a manner similar to those when the pet was present, correlations between Burke Dementia Scale score and socialization variables also were calculated for the control session. Significant correlations for frequency of smiles and verbalization and duration of smiles, verbalization, and temporal response occurred (see Table 13.2).

Split-plot ANOVA was used to examine whether the amount of increase in socialization in the presence of the therapy dog was related to severity

TABLE 13.2   Correlations Between Socialization Variables
and Burke Dementia Scale Scores

Variable	Control	Experimental
Frequency Variables		
Leans toward	0.16	−0.03
Smiles	−0.43*	−0.54*
Tactile contact	—	−0.31
Look	0.01	−0.40*
Physical warmth	—	0.43*
Praise	0.20	−0.69*
Verbalization	−0.50*	−0.37
Duration Variables		
Leans toward	0.16	−0.11
Smiles	−0.60*	−0.40
Tactile contact	—	−0.29
Look	−0.04	−0.45*
Temporal response	0.43*	−0.25
Verbalization	−0.53*	−0.46*

NOTE: Higher scores on the Burke Dementia Scale indicate greater impairment.
$*p < .05.$

of the participant's dementia. Participants were divided into three equal groups by severity of dementia. A significant treatment by group effect was found for praise only, $F (1, 19) = 12.37$, $p < .01$. Those least impaired showed a significantly greater increase in praise frequency during the experimental versus control session.

Using repeated measures ANOVA, no significant interaction effects were found for blood pressure, mean blood pressure, pulse, or peripheral skin temperature. There was a greater increase in skin temperature from baseline in the experimental session than in the control session (an increase of 2.70° and 1.82°, respectively); this difference, however, did not reach significance.

Discussion

The presence of the therapy dog enhanced nonverbal communication as shown by increases in looks, smiles, tactile contact, and physical warmth. Looks and smiles may be considered indicators of pleasure and interest, whereas touch is suggested as an important facet of communication. Touch may fulfill many functions, such as comfort and contact with reality, and has been suggested as a necessary element of mental and physical health (Weiss, 1979). It is noteworthy that touch had a zero occurrence in the sessions without the therapy dog. The opportunity for leans toward responses was limited because the investigator and dog's proximity to the participant did not require leans.

There were no significant differences in overall verbalizations when the dog was present; more praise, however, did occur when the dog was present. This finding could be interpreted as an increase in communication of positive feelings or intent. Anecdotally, it was observed that participants made responses that could be described as comforting or might indicate bonding with another when the pet was present and that these statements were directed to the pet. Examples of these statements include, "You understand, don't you?" and "That's a nice dog, you're a good dog, yes you are." Such statements are consistent with Netting, Wilson, and New's (1987) supposition that pets may allow the older person opportunities for other roles such as a caregiver, confidant, or companion.

The findings of this study are congruent with previous research regarding the positive effects of a therapy dog on socialization during short-term interactions. Both the current study and research by Kongable and colleagues (1989) found significant increases in overall socialization for participants with AD in conditions in which the pet was present. Despite many methodological differences between the current study and that of Furstenberg, Rhodes, and Powell (1988), both studies demonstrated a significant increase in social interaction for participants with AD when a pet was present. Findings showing more overall socialization when the pet was present are generally consistent with earlier studies (e.g., Brunmeier et al., 1986; Buelt et al., 1985) that examined the effect of pets on socialization in other populations of older persons.

Although there were significant increases in socialization behaviors by the person with AD, it is likely that the increase would be greater in a natural setting rather than in the experimental conditions of this study. In this study, after the initial introduction to the dog, the investigator no longer drew the participant's attention to the dog. In a pet therapy situation, encouragement and reminders about the pet's presence would likely increase socialization with the pet and therapist. Moreover, the resident and dog would be free to move around the room; lack of movement was a constraint of this study related to placement of the video camera and the physiological monitoring instruments. As expected, several indicators of socialization decreased as the severity of dementia increased. Except for the variable frequency of praise, there were no differences by level of dementia for changes in the amount of socialization in the experimental versus control situation. It was projected that those with severe impairment might be less able to interact with the dog. The finding that level of impairment did not significantly affect the outcome might mean that a therapy dog may activate a more basic form of communication or socialization for which those with greater impairment may participate.

Indicators of a relaxation response were not different between experimental and control conditions. Participants' greater alertness (evidenced by a higher occurrence of looks) and possibly increased activity associated with petting the dog may have offset a relaxation effect (Schuelke et al., 1991-1992). The majority of participants either were taking medications or had a medical condition with the potential to affect circulatory response, which may have attenuated the physiological responses. It is unknown how these mediators may have affected the socialization variables, but because a within-participants design was used in which each participant participated in both experimental and control conditions, the use of medications would not have biased the results. Hulbert, Hulbert, and Lonn (1985) also reported no heart rate changes in older participants when they petted a friendly dog.

Similarly, no changes in blood pressure were found by Schuelke et al. (1991-1992) in individuals with hypertension, although a significant increase in skin temperature did occur. Conflicting findings between Schuelke and colleague's research and the current study regarding skin temperature changes may be related to age differences in the participants involved in these two studies. The mean age of participants in Schuelke and colleagues' research was 50.3 years of age, whereas the mean age of the participants in the current study was 77.9 years of age. Another difference that may have contributed to conflicting findings was the use of a dog familiar to the participants in the Schuelke et al. study. Significantly greater increases in skin temperature occurred when participants petted their own dog compared with when they petted an unknown dog. Perhaps greater increases in skin temperature would have been found in the current study if the participants had been more familiar with the therapy dog.

Videotaping was used in this study. A concern prior to the study was that the camera might affect the participants' behavior. This concern proved to be unfounded because only two individuals asked about the camera and subsequently made no further note of it.

Continued research that focuses on the therapeutic benefits of pets in promoting increased socialization and stress reduction for those with AD is needed. Future investigations examining which pet characteristics are associated with higher amounts of socialization, comparing the effect of pets on socialization in group versus individual settings, and examining optimal length of interaction between the person and the pet may be useful. It has been well documented that pets provide other services for human beings beyond that of companionship. Research to determine alternative roles of pets for persons with AD is warranted.

Studies with larger numbers of participants are needed to further test the impact of pets on stress response. The number of participants in this study did not allow for analysis of the effect of cardiovascular medication or conditions on physiological variables. Using more than one type of stress measure, such as an observational measure, also may be helpful.

The findings of this study suggest that pet therapy is one intervention that should be promoted and implemented for persons with AD. Psychological needs for which pet therapy should be recommended include the need for sensory input, role enactment, comfort, and communication through touch. Pet therapy appears to be a stimulus that matches the level of cognitive impairment for this group of individuals. The use of pet therapy with persons with AD provides an easily implemented intervention. It fills a basic need for communication as well as for physical contact.

References

American Psychiatric Association. (1987). *Diagnostic and statistical manual of mental disorders* (3rd ed.). Washington, DC: Author.

Baun, M., Bergstrom, N., Langston, N., & Thoma, L. (1984). Physiological effects of human/companion animal bonding. *Nursing Research, 33,* 126-129.

Bern, R., & Levy, M. (1983). The arterial system. In R. Bern & M. Levy (Eds.), *Physiology* (pp. 504-517). St. Louis, MO: C. V. Mosby.

Brody, E., Lawton, M., & Liebowitz, B. (1984). Senile dementia: Public policy and adequate institutional care. *American Journal of Public Health, 74,* 1381-1383.

Brunmeier, C., McArthur, M., Baun, M., & Bergstrom, N. (1986). *The effect of a dog on the social interaction of mentally impaired institutionalized elderly.* Unpublished manuscript, University of Nebraska Medical Center, College of Nursing, Omaha.

Buelt, M., Bergstrom, N., Baun, M., & Langston, N. (1985). Facilitating social interaction among institutionalized elderly through use of a companion dog. [Abstract]. *Proceedings from the 1985 Annual Delta Society Conference, 2,* 62.

Daubenmire, J., White, J., Heinzerling, K., Ashton, C., & Searles, S. (1977). *Synchronics: A notation for the quantitative and qualitative description of presenting behaviors* (RF 760059). Columbus: Ohio State University Research Foundation.

Fritz, C. L., Farver, T. B., Hart, L. A., & Kass, P. H. (1996). Companion animals and the psychological health of Alzheimer's patients' caregivers. *Psychological Reports, 78,* 467-481.

Fritz, C. L., Farver, T. B., Kass, P. H., & Hart, L. A. (1995). Association with companion animals and the expression of noncognitive symptoms in Alzheimer's patients. *Journal of Nervous and Mental Disease, 183*(7), 459-463.

Furstenberg, F., Rhodes, P., & Powell, S. (1988). Short-term value of pets. *American Journal of Nursing, 88*(2), 157.

Grossberg, J., & Alf, E. (1985). Interaction with pet dogs: Effects on human cardiovascular response. *Journal of the Delta Society, 2,* 20-27.

Hall, G., & Buckwalter, K. (1987). Progressively lowered stress threshold: A conceptual model for care of adults with Alzheimer's disease. *Archives of Psychiatric Nursing, 1,* 429-436.

Haycox, J. A. (1984). A simple, reliable clinical behavioral scale for assessing demented patients. *Journal of Clinical Psychiatry, 45,* 23-24.

Hulbert, R., Hulbert, T., & Lonn, S. (1985). *Heart rate response to touch: One aspect of the person-pet relationship.* Unpublished manuscript, University of Nebraska, Lincoln.

Katzman, R., & Jackson, J. (1991). Alzheimer's disease: Basic and clinical advances. *Journal of the American Geriatrics Society, 39*(5), 516-525.

Kogan, K., & Gordon, B. (1975). Interpersonal behavior constructs: A revised approach to defining dyadic interaction style. *Psychological Reports, 36,* 835-846.

Kongable, L., Buckwalter, K. C., & Stolley, J. (1989). The effects of pet therapy on the social behavior of institutionalized Alzheimer's clients. *Archives of Psychiatric Nursing, 3,* 191-198.

Kongable, L., Stolley, J., & Buckwalter, K. C. (1990). Pet therapy for Alzheimer's patients: A survey. *Journal of Long Term Care Administration, 18*(3), 17-21.

Lee, V. (1991). Language changes and Alzheimer's disease: A literature review. *Journal of Gerontological Nursing, 17*(1), 16-20.

Mace, N., & Rabins, P. (1991). *The 36-hour day.* Baltimore: Johns Hopkins University Press.

Netting, F., Wilson, C., & New, J. (1987). The human-animal bond: Implications for practice. *Social Work, 32,* 60-64.

Schuelke, S., Trask, B., Wallace, C., Baun, M., Bergstrom, N., & McCabe, B. (1991-1992). Physiological effects of the use of a companion animal dog as a cue to relaxation in diagnosed hypertensives. *Latham Letter, 8*(1), 14-17.

U.S. Congress. (1987). *Losing a million minds: Confronting the tragedy of Alzheimer's disease and other dementias* (Publication No. OTA-BA-323). Washington, DC: Government Printing Office.)

Weiss, S. (1979). The language of touch. *Nursing Research, 28,* 76-80.

PART V

Human Growth and Development: Age-Specific Quality of Life Outcomes

Cindy C. Wilson
Dennis C. Turner

Quality of life (QL) is applicable to all ages, conditions, and abilities. In this section, Melson responds to the call for a theoretical framework for understanding children's development and considers the subjective symptoms, feelings, and well-being relevant to children's ability to meet developmental challenges. She then presents hypotheses against which the literature may be compared with the framework and identifies research gaps.

A more specific assessment of an element of QL (i.e., well-being) is made by Bodmer as she focuses on the relationship of pet ownership and well-being of adolescents who report few familiar resources. Pet owners tended to have higher levels of well-being but also higher levels of familial resources than did nonowners. No moderating effect of pet ownership on relationship between few familial resources and well-being was seen.

Interest in QL as a conceptual framework has been stimulated by ethical and financial considerations associated with an aging population and the concomitant increase in chronic illness. QL, however, is applicable to all ages, conditions, and abilities. Improving QL is a key ingredient in normal growth and development and in therapeutic interventions, as well as in rehabilitation programs. It is as important to an individual with good health and many resources as it is to the person who is hearing impaired or the individual with low self-esteem.

The Role of Companion Animals in Human Development 14

Gail F. Melson

Abstract

This chapter considers the role of companion animals in children's development, with emphasis on how companion animals may affect quality of life for children. Because companion animals must be available to children to exert influence on their development, evidence for availability of companion animals is first reviewed. Then, a framework, derived from existing theories on human development, is applied to examine quality of life in children's development. The framework is used to generate hypotheses about how companion animals might affect children's quality of life. Existing literature is examined as it bears on each of these hypotheses, and directions for future research are suggested. The major goals of this chapter are (a) to link research and theory related to human-companion animal relationships; (b) to apply broad, "mainstream" ideas about children's development to consideration of the role of companion animals; and (c) to suggest a programmatic, theory-based blueprint for research, one that points to future areas of inquiry as well as organizes past research.

Throughout the world, companion animals and children live together, each developing and changing, together part of a family system, which, in turn, is embedded in the multiple environments of neighborhood, community, and society. In some parts of the world, children are more likely to dwell with pets than with their grandparents and, in many cases, their siblings or even their fathers (Melson & Yu, 1996). What role do companion animals play in human development, particularly, in the development of children? How might that role or (more likely) roles affect children's quality of life?

Despite long-standing recognition of the close ties between people of all ages and companion animals, an answer to these questions is not available because we are at the beginning of scientific inquiry. The goal of this chapter is to suggest a framework for understanding how interactions with companion animals may affect children's quality of life (QL). To do this, QL is first defined as applied to children's development. A framework is then described that places the study of companion animals within the theoretical traditions of contemporary psychology. From this framework, hypotheses are derived concerning the role that pets and other animals may play in children's quality of life. Existing research is reviewed as it bears on these hypotheses. Where research is lacking, directions for a future research agenda are suggested.

Availability of Companion Animals in Children's Lives

First, what do researchers know about the availability of companion animals to children? This is an important first question, because animals are unlikely to affect children if they are not accessible to them. Indirect, mediated effects, as occur when parents and others tell children stories about animals or when children view media images of companion animals, should not be discounted (McCrindle & Odendaal, 1994). In North America and Europe, pets are found in the majority of households with children (Rowan, 1992). There are significant variations, however, by child, family, and community characteristics. Much of the available information on pet ownership rates comes from convenience samples or samples drawn from limited populations. There are virtually no systematic, national, or cross-national data on pet ownership, a serious shortcoming. Therefore, generalizations about companion animal ownership should be interpreted with caution.

Nonetheless, some consistent patterns do emerge from the existing data.

1. *Families with children are more likely to own companion animals than are families without children* (Salmon & Salmon, 1983). These ownership rates tend to be high. For example, 88% of British university students recalled childhood pet ownership (Paul & Serpell, 1992).

2. *Families with either very young children or teenagers are less likely to own pets than are families with school-age children.* For example, Rost and Hartmann (1994) found that 80% of fourth graders in Hesse, Germany, currently or recently owned a pet, a figure comparable with that found for a sample (Melson, 1988) of midwestern U.S. elementary school children (70%), Kidd and Kidd's (1985, 1990a, 1990b) California samples (90%), and Bryant's (1985) California sample of grade school children (90%). In contrast, 44% of preschoolers were in families with companion animals (Melson, 1988).

3. *Multiple pet ownership is also common.* Bryant (1985) reported that 60% of her sample of California 10-year olds had two or more pets. In a study of the role of pets for young children making the transition to public school, 60% of these pet-owning families had multiple pets (Melson & Schwartz, 1994).

4. *Many child, family, and environmental factors influence pet ownership.* Pet ownership appears more likely when children have no siblings or few siblings (Melson, 1988; Rost & Hartmann, 1994) or live in rural versus urban areas or in houses versus apartments (Rost & Hartmann, 1994). Still, across a variety of settings and family configurations, reported ranges of pet ownership suggest that the majority of children in Western industrialized nations are living with companion animals.

Pet ownership is undoubtedly the major way in which companion animals are available to children, but other modes of direct exposure are receiving increasing attention. Companion animals owned by others in the neighborhood or by extended family are potentially available to children (Bryant, 1985). Increasingly, classrooms and day care centers have resident pets. Perhaps the first item on a future research agenda should be comprehensive description of the variety of settings in which children regularly encounter companion animals.

Assessment of exposure to companion animals is important because it describes a necessary condition for assessing influence. Mere availability of companion animals tells us little about their impact on children. Studies of children and companion animals have consistently found that pet ownership (i.e., the presence of companion animals within the home) is not related in any significant way to measures of children's development (Melson, 1988; Poresky & Hendrix, 1990). Not surprisingly, it is the quality of the relationship, not simply interaction opportunities, that is significant.

A Framework for Understanding Children's Quality of Life

Although there is disagreement on a conceptual definition (Aaronson, 1989), Wilson (1994) offers a useful definition of "quality of life (QL)" as "clinically relevant aspects of subjective symptoms, feelings, and well-being" (p. 4). In general, the QL construct has been applied only to adults, particularly older persons and those with acute or chronic illnesses. A major problem with definitions derived from the latter half of the life span is their failure to give emphasis to developmental change, which must be central to any definition of children's QL. Despite this, QL provides a useful umbrella construct that with some modifications can be applied across the life span. Such a life span focus permits examination of relations with companion animals as "flexible affiliations" that change as individuals age (Wilson & Netting, 1987).

Quality of life, as applied to children's development, needs to take into account the developmental challenges or tasks that confront children as part of typical developmental sequences. Thus, QL for children may be defined as *the subjective symptoms, feelings, and well-being relevant to the child's ability to meet developmental challenges.* Several important components to this definition are (a) an emphasis on the child's *perception* or interpretation of reality, reflecting the view that children (like people of all ages) construct their reality and that their perceptions of their well-being are a more important predictor of outcomes than an outsider's assessment; and (b) an emphasis on QL as *relative* to the different development needs of children at different periods of development. Thus, the same prompt responsiveness and nurturance of a caregiver that reassures a 2-year-old may thwart the autonomy needs of a 12-year-old.

Erikson's (1963) life cycle stage theory is a useful guide to identify developmental challenges. To better understand those factors that may influence children's ability to meet developmental challenges, a second theoretical perspective is needed. Ecological systems theory (Bronfenbrenner, 1979, 1986) describes the influence of multiple aspects of children's environments and relationships on their ability to meet developmental challenges. These two theoretical perspectives provide a fruitful framework within which to organize an understanding of how companion animals help (or hinder) children in meeting developmental challenges and hence affect their QL.

From Erikson's (1963) theory, four central developmental challenges of childhood emerge—trust, autonomy, industry, and identity. Each challenge lays the foundation for the next, although all may remain active throughout childhood. *Trust* refers to the infant's reassurance that the world is a welcoming, rather than a hostile, place; *autonomy* to the preschooler's need to move out from the cocoon of trusting relationships to explore independently; *industry* to the school-age child's drive to master skills; and *identity* to the adolescent's search for an independent adult self.

In articulating the ecological systems perspective, Bronfenbrenner (1979) first emphasizes that children's development is profoundly affected by what he calls the *microsystems* of their environment, that is, the face-to-face settings in which children develop—most typically, home, school, and peer group. Not surprisingly, this is where most research on children and companion animals has focused, in the realm of direct encounters between children and (usually) their pets. Second, the connections among these microsystems (what Bronfenbrenner calls the *mesosystem*) exert influence on development; as an example, he argues that children develop more optimally when values at home and at school are concordant rather than discordant. To apply this mesosystem construct to the study of children and companion animals, one might examine how interactions with companion animals in one setting (e.g., the home) are related to such interactions in another setting (i.e., with a classroom pet or neighborhood animals)—or, more broadly, how children's attachments to their pets at home affect their functioning in school or in their peer interactions. Third, environmental influences may affect children indirectly through their effects on parents, peers, or teachers. This environmental dimension Bronfenbrenner calls the *exosystem*. As an example, "family-friendly" work conditions may help parents be more effective caregivers and thereby indirectly influence the child's development. There may be fruitful applications of this exosystem construct to the study of relationships between children and companion animals. A parent's attachment to a companion animal may indirectly affect the child through the pet's impact on the parent. Finally, Bronfenbrenner suggests that overarching environmental

Table 14.1   A Conceptual Framework for Examining Companion Animals in Relation to Children's Quality of Life

Developmental Challenge	Microsystem	Mesosystem	Exosystem	Macrosystem
Basic trust	CA as secure base	CA attachment in relation to human attachments	CA as support for parent to provide responsivity	Cultural value of animal as attachment figure
Autonomy initiative	CA as playmate	CA playmate in relation to human playmates	Neighborhood or community influences on CA availability	Cultural value of animals as play partners
Industry	CA as learning aid	Relation between CA and other learning aids	CA effects on learning environment (e.g., teacher morale)	Cultural value of CA as learning opportunity
Identity	CA as support	Relation between CA and other supports for identity exploration	CA as support for parents, peers	Cultural value of CA as part of adolescent identity exploration

NOTE: CA = companion animal.

influences such as cultural values, the *macrosystem* level, permeate all aspects of the environment. This construct draws attention to cultural variation in how relationships between children and companion animals are structured and given meaning.

The integration of an Eriksonian developmental perspective with a "Bronfenbrennerian" environmental perspective suggests that the sequence of typically occurring developmental challenges that unfold as children mature should be examined, as well as the role of multiple environmental influences affecting how children respond to these challenges. Both Erikson and Bronfenbrenner acknowledge that the child's own genetic makeup makes an important contribution to how the child meets developmental challenges. Even when children face the same developmental challenges within the same constellation of environmental influences, there will nonetheless be considerable individual variability.

The framework proposed has these advantages for advancing understanding of the role of companion animals in children's development: (a) It takes account of both developmental change and multiple environmental influences; (b) it integrates research and theory on children's relationships with animals into thinking about the impact of other relationships on children's development, thus applying psychological and sociological constructs to a new field; and (c) it permits application of the QL construct, thereby facilitating a life span approach to QL. Table 14.1 presents an overview of this conceptual framework applied to the role of companion animals in children's development. In short, the proposed framework suggests potential companion animal influences at each of four environmental levels on children's ability to meet developmental challenges.

Using this framework to organize current research knowledge on the role of companion animals in children's development reveals a concentration of studies in a few "cells." Such a conceptual organization of current literature can help illustrate gaps in knowledge and research questions that need to be addressed. The following sections describe four developmental challenges—trust, autonomy, industry, and identity. Hypotheses are derived to suggest how companion animals may be important for each challenge at four environmental levels of influence—microsystem, mesosystem, exosystem, and macrosystem.

The Developmental Challenge of Basic Trust

Erikson (1963) suggests that the first developmental challenge for children is basic trust, the reassurance that one's needs will be met, leading the child to the belief in the world as a benign and hence interesting, rather than threatening, place. There is considerable evidence, organized within the related theoretical tradition called attachment theory (Bretherton, 1985), that basic trust stems from the microsystem influence of responsive caregiving, leading the child to form a secure attachment relationship with one or more significant individuals. Thus, security of attachment is the hallmark of an infant's QL. Without security of attachment, the infant's cognitive and physical development is compromised, as well as the ability to form trusting relationships. Secure attachment relationships, providing reassurance of the child's safety and worthiness, continue to be important as the child matures.

Research suggests that children form multiple attachments to the significant individuals in their world, generally mother, father, and sibling (Waters, Vaughn, Posada, & Kondo-Ikemura, 1995). It appears that a range of individuals in the child's microsystems can provide responsive care. For example, Stewart (1983) has demonstrated that older siblings can provide the responsiveness that reassures infants and contributes to their basic trust. When pets are present in young children's lives, do they contribute to the children's sense of security? If so, how might they do so? Because the reassurance provided by a secure attachment continues to be important through childhood, as it is reactivated during times of stress, do older children also turn to companion animals for such reassurance? These questions suggest the first hypothesis:

> *Companion animals promote the quality of life of children by contributing to their sense of basic trust.*

There is considerable evidence that as early as age 3 (if not younger), children characteristically establish a differentiated, nonsubstitutable relationship with the pet, a relationship that provides emotional assurance in times of stress. Even quite young children form strong emotional attachments to companion animals (Melson, Peet, & Sparks, 1991). For example, 95% of the 300 children ages 3 to 13 in the San Francisco area interviewed by Kidd and Kidd (1985) reported mutuality of love with their pets. But do such attachments provide the secure base (to use Bowlby's [1969] term) that promotes basic trust? This is less clear. With very young children, it should be possible to see this activated under conditions of moderate stress, such as in the Strange Situation, the most common assessment of security of attachment. In this assessment, the young child is observed in a playroom first with the attachment figure, usually the child's mother, then with an adult stranger, alone, again with the stranger, and finally, reuniting with the attachment figure. The child's ability to be reassured by the attachment figure, especially during reunion, and to use the attachment figure as a "secure base" from which to venture out to explore the playroom and get acquainted with the stranger provides a window into the child's sense of basic trust in this relationship. A study examining the child with the pet in the Strange Situation has not been undertaken but might be illuminating. Does the presence of the child's pet reassure the child during separations from human attachment figures or provide a secure base from which to explore? Because the presence of a companion animal is effective in decreasing the physiological arousal of children (Friedmann, Katcher, Thomas, Lynch, & Messent, 1983), it is plausible that a companion animal may serve as a source of reassurance during stress.

Reports from somewhat older school-age children provide convergent evidence that some children turn to companion animals in times of stress for reassurance. The majority of the German fourth graders in Rost and Hartmann's (1994) study reported turning to their pets when they were sad, and nearly half preferred the company of their pets to that of other children. Similarly, in Indiana, when pet-owning 5-year-olds were asked to whom they would turn when feeling sad, 25% of them spontaneously mentioned their pets. Ten percent mentioned their pets when asked to whom they would turn when feeling afraid (Melson & Schwarz, 1994). Covert, Whiren, Keith, and Nelson (1985) found that 75% of Michigan youngsters ages 10 to 14 indicated that they turned to their pets when feeling upset. Finally, in Bryant's (1985) interviews with 10-year-olds, 13% of the children spontaneously mentioned turning to pets when feeling stress. These wide variations in percentages may reflect differences in research methodology, such as sample characteristics, question wording, and mode of administration, as well as confounding variables such as type of pet. Nonetheless, it is clear that a minority of children from preschool through adolescence use pets as attachment figures for reassurance in times of insecurity.

These findings raise further questions. Which children are most likely to use pets for reassurance? One study found, not surprisingly, that 5-year-olds who reported playing with their pets more and who felt their pets really cared for them were more likely to spontaneously mention their pets as a source of support when the children felt sad, angry, or happy. Moreover, those children who reported more emotional closeness and support from their pets were less likely to be described by their mothers or fathers as anxious and withdrawn (Melson, Windecker-Nelson, & Schwarz, 1997). In some circumstances, however, does turning to a pet for reassurance make the use of human attachments less likely? For example, Bryant (1985) found that those 10-year-olds who often sought reassurance from their pets were functioning less optimally 4 years later, showing less cooperation with peers, than were children who had been less dependent on their pets. When does the use of companion animals for reassurance help and when does it interfere with the child's ability to meet other developmental challenges, such as autonomy, independence, and the establishment of multiple relationships with humans? These questions can be answered by examining the qualities of the child-companion animal relationship in the context of the child's multiple relationships with humans, rather than in isolation from other relationships.

It is important to recognize that attachment relationships may increase children's stress and anxiety even as they reassure them. Bryant's (1987) interviews with children ages 7, 10, and 14 document that children were often anxious about the well-being of their pets and on occasion felt aggression and anger toward them. Their descriptions of their relationships with their pets contained both positive and negative elements (Bryant, 1990).

The role of companion animals as indirect supports for children's basic trust has received no attention to date. This exosystem influence suggests that the relationships that caregivers and parents have with companion animals might affect the attachment relationships these adults or older children establish with children. For example, by reducing stress in parents, do companion animals thereby enable them to be more responsive to children? The ability of companion animals to reduce physiological arousal in adults also has been well established (Friedmann, Locker, & Lockwood, 1993) but as yet not linked to family interactions.

The Developmental Challenge of Autonomy

A second developmental challenge is to achieve mastery over the physical and social environment through the development of autonomy, exploration, and initiative. Reassured about their own basic safety through secure attachments, children then feel free to explore their gradually expanding world through play, to develop new relationships, and to test the growing capacities of their maturing bodies and brains. This suggests a second hypothesis:

Companion animals promote quality of life in children by facilitating play, exploration, and independence.

There is ample evidence that children perceive their companion animals as play partners. This is more likely during middle childhood than during adolescence or early childhood (Kidd & Kidd, 1985). Melson et al. (1991) found that second- and fifth-grade midwestern U.S. children described their relationship with their pets predominantly as play. Similarly, Rost and Hartmann (1994) reported that a majority of the German fourth graders they studied indicated that they played, talked with, or were affectionate with their pets daily. In Bryant's (1985) interviews with California 10-year-olds, themes of play and companionship predominated in answers to the question, "What makes your pet a special friend?"

Although researchers know that children's interactions with pets often center around play (Kidd & Kidd, 1985), there is need for more detailed information about the content and quality of these play interactions. How cognitively complex is this play? For example, children's play with peers may be categorized into levels of complexity, with sociodramatic or pretend play considered most complex and hence more conducive to cognitive development through enriched use of language, opportunities to take the perspective of others, and extended problem-solving experiences. A psychoanalytic perspective on play suggests that play provides a safe arena for the child to act out fears or repressed urges (Shell, 1993). To what extent might such themes or levels of complexity exist in children's play with companion animals?

The study of children's play with companion animals may also be linked to their play with humans. For example, to what extent does play with a companion animal serve as a social lubricant to the play of two or more children? There is evidence that the presence of service dogs increases social interaction for children with disabilities (Mader, Hart, & Bergin, 1989). Would the presence of a companion animal increase social interaction for children without disabilities who are socially rejected or isolated? When a companion animal is present as two children play together, how does the animal change the content and quality of the child-child interaction?

To answer these questions, we as researchers need to move beyond surveys of children and their parents to more in-depth ethological observations of play behaviors involving children and their companion animals. Basic descriptive data on the quality of child-companion animal play in different settings are needed. Experimental studies could then be conducted to examine changes in child-child interaction when an animal is present versus absent, or in play with a child versus in proximity to the child.

The Developmental Challenge of Industry

The elementary school or preadolescent years are described by Erikson (1963) as focused on the developmental challenge of learning skills, of being industrious in the sense of deriving pleasure from completing significant tasks. The child's felt success in this area is mirrored in feelings of self-competence, a sense of being "good at" learning things. Influences on meeting the challenge of industry stem not only from success at previous developmental challenges but also from a variety of other environmental influences. On the microsystem level, the role of authoritative parenting (combining warmth, firmness, and acceptance; Baumrind, 1973), peer acceptance (being liked by other children; Coie, Dodge, & Coppotelli, 1982), and moderately challenging problem solving (Siegler, 1983) has been well documented. Mesosystem influences on meeting the challenge of industry have also been found, for example, the critical links between family and school. When parents are knowledgeable about the learning tasks their children are likely to encounter at school and endorse the skills necessary to master these tasks, they can more effectively support their child's learning (Okagaki & Sternberg, 1993). Exosystem influences operating on parents, teachers, and schools to indirectly affect children's learning also have received extensive attention. As an example, school policy may create conflicting demands on teacher time and decrease focused attention on the child's learning. Finally, macrosystem influences have been documented (Stevenson & Lee, 1990), showing that cultural beliefs shared by parents and teachers about how children learn powerfully affect children's school achievement.

The role of companion animals in fostering learning skills and self-competence warrants investigation on all environmental levels. This leads to the third hypothesis:

Companion animals promote quality of life in children by aiding in learning and in acquisition of self-competence.

One aspect of learning is the acquisition of knowledge about animals, both companion animals and other animals. A second aspect is the use of companion animals to facilitate learning skills in other domains. For example, parents often report that they acquire pets to help teach their children responsibility and caring for others. Teachers use classroom pets not only to impart knowledge about animals and their care but also as indirect aids to learning—as reinforcers, diversions, or relaxants.

On the microsystem level, direct effects of companion animals can be measured by examining the impact of classroom animals and special curricula (Antonelli, Beck, Bennett, Bradley, Freeman, Fricke, Grippi, Ketterer, & Sokoloff, 1991) designed to teach children about both animals and human-animal relationships (for example, humane education). In a well-controlled intervention study, Ascione (1992) demonstrated that a school humane education program resulted in more positive attitudes by fourth graders toward both companion and noncompanion animals, as well as in more empathy directed toward humans.

There is little systematic evidence, however, that classroom pets enhance learning either about the animals themselves or about other subjects. Well-controlled intervention studies like that of Ascione (1992) are needed to determine what forms of classroom involvement with animals may enhance what types of learning. Moreover, if effects are found, process-oriented research is then urgently needed to examine what processes of teacher, child, and animal behavior underlie the effects found. For example, it is possible that the presence of a classroom pet or even a fish tank may reduce distraction or tension and improve concentration, thus, indirectly supporting learning. Or it may be that certain interactive opportunities, such as time to visit with or handle a classroom pet, may have a calming effect on highly active and distracted children. There is anecdotal evidence from educators of such effects, but documentation is lacking.

Within the microsystem of the family, there is a paucity of evidence concerning what companion animals might be teaching children or how the presence of companion animals might affect learning. Do companion animals promote responsibility and nurturing in children, as many parents believe? There is little evidence on this question. A secondary analysis of records of daily activity for a nationally representative sample of families with children from ages 3 to 18 was recently completed (Melson & Yu, 1996). According to the children's own reports (or if they were under 5, their parents' reports), pet-owning children did not do more household chores or spend more time caring for others, such as younger siblings. They did little pet care, which, along with other aspects of household work, was predominantly done by mothers.

The role pets play in influencing children's acquisition of responsibility or empathy will likely vary by child and family factors. Take, for example, the age of the child. Relationships with pets appear to be associated with aspects of development in different ways, depending on the age of the child. Bryant (1985) found that 10-year-olds who report "having more intimate talks with pets" showed higher empathy, more acceptance of individual differences, and more competitive attitudes. The 7-year-olds she interviewed who reported having more intimate talks with pets, however, showed *lower* empathy, *less* acceptance of individual differences, and *less* competitive attitudes. Similarly, in studies of Indiana schoolchildren, attachment to one's pet was associated with greater empathy and more positive self-concept among 5- to 6-year-olds but not 7- to 8- or 10- to 11-year-olds (Melson et al., 1991). These findings underscore the importance of considering developmental change because even during the period of industry, links between relationships with companion animals and important outcomes such as responsibility and empathy vary by age.

The Challenge of Identity

Erikson (1963) suggested that the exploration of identity typically begins in adolescence when the child must consider what sort of adult to become and how that future adult relates to the child that was. The role that companion animals might play in the identity process has not been considered, and it might seem implausible to suggest any. But a speculative final hypothesis may be advanced:

> *Companion animals play a role in identity exploration and achievement through their ability to provide a nonjudgmental "audience."*

Erikson (1963) suggests that identity exploration is facilitated by discussion. Both heated exchanges with parents and long rap sessions with friends may serve the function of clarifying the adolescent's thoughts. Studies (Grotevant & Cooper, 1985) suggest that warm, accepting parents best support their teenager's identity exploration. Perhaps the warm, accepting presence of a nonjudgmental companion animal may provide one of the contexts in which adolescents can explore ideas and feelings freely.

Studies that extend this inquiry might pose the following questions: (a) What types of relationships do adolescents have with companion animals?

What are the characteristics of (undoubtedly a small minority of) adolescents who rely on companion animals as confidants and discussion partners? (b) How does the presence of a companion animal modify adolescents' interactions with friends and with family? (c) Is the quality of the relationship between adolescent and companion animal related to measures of identity, and how does that relationship differ in different families and for different children? At the exosystem level, how does the parent's or friend's relationship with a companion animal affect his or her ability to support the adolescent's identity exploration?

In summary, placing the study of children and companion animals within broader theoretical frameworks advances the field in several ways: (a) It organizes existing knowledge, (b) it illuminates neglected areas of inquiry, (c) it helps relate findings to other influences on development, and (d) it suggests a programmatic approach to future research.

To enhance knowledge of the potential role that companion animals may play in enhancing QL aspects of daily living, eight specific suggestions are presented:

1. *Build developmental change into the study of children and companion animals.* Longitudinal studies can help both capture how earlier relationships with companion animals affect later development and disentangle cause-effect relations from correlational findings. Short-term longitudinal designs can take advantage of naturally occurring developmental transitions. For example, young children's transition into public school or adjustment to the birth of a sibling might be examined by assessing relationships with companion animals before and after the transition.

2. *Consider the role of companion animals in context.* This chapter has emphasized that relationships with companion animals occur in the context of other, human relationships and in interrelated settings of home, school, peer group, and neighborhood. With a few exceptions (cf. Bryant, 1985), the child-companion animal relationship has been viewed in isolation. Instead, one must study the importance of animals for children *in relation* to children's human relationships.

3. *Examine indirect or exosystem influences of companion animals on children.* The relationships that parents, teachers, and friends have with animals may affect their interactions with children and, through this indirect pathway, affect children's development. Analogously, settings that provide animal companionship or visitation may exert beneficial effects on groups such as persons who are older, who are chronically ill, and who have emotional illness, in part through their effects on the human caregivers in these settings.

4. *Attend to cultural variation in the relationship between children and companion animals.* There are rich anthropological descriptions of the relationships between children and animals (Savishinsky, 1974) in various cultures, but this work has not informed psychological studies. Systematic cross-cultural comparisons are urgently needed. Cultures weave myths and tales that link children with animals, from Romulus and Remus to "Where the Wild Things Are," and these cultural templates may affect the type, frequency, and quality of children's relationships with companion animals.

5. *Conduct more observational and experimental studies.* Previous research has relied on survey and interview methods. These approaches need to be supplemented with more basic observation of children with companion animals. In addition, well-controlled intervention studies are needed.

6. *Use existing research paradigms.* As noted, established methodologies such as the Strange Situation to assess security of attachment, or one of several well-established observational coding schemes for categorizing children's play, can be modified to examine the role of companion animals.

7. *Consider the specificity of environmental influences.* Researchers need to move beyond asking, "How do companion animals influence children's development?" to asking, in keeping with Wach's theory of environmental specificity (Wachs & Gruen, 1982), the far more sophisticated question, "For what children under what conditions do companion animals influence which aspects of development?"

8. *Recognize the possibility of negative as well as positive outcomes associated with companion animals.* As noted, relationships with companion animals (like all relationships) may give rise to negative emotions, may increase stress (Bryant, 1990), and may impede healthy development. Childhood cruelty to animals may be an early marker of later delinquency (Ascione, 1994; Kellert & Felthous, 1985). We need to study the conditions under which such negative outcomes occur as vigorously as we study the benefits of companion animals.

In conclusion, a programmatic body of research well grounded in developmental theory and methods does not yet exist to inform our knowledge of the role of companion animals for children's development, but its outlines may be drawn from major theories such as Erikson's psychosocial theory and Bronfenbrenner's ecological theory.

References

Aaronson, N. K. (1989). Quality of life assessment in clinical trials: Methodological issues. *Controlled Clinical Trials, 10,* 195-208.

Antonelli, M., Beck, A. M., Bennett, E., Bradley, E., Freeman, C. C., Fricke, S., Grippi, B., Ketterer, D., & Sokoloff, H. J. (1991). *Pets and me: A thematic learning experience built on the relationships between people and animals.* Philadelphia: University of Pennsylvania Press.

Ascione, F. R. (1992). Enhancing children's attitudes about the humane treatment of animals: Generalizations to human-directed empathy. *Anthrozoös, 5,* 176-191.

Ascione, F. R. (1994). Children who are cruel to animals: A review of research and implication for developmental psychopathology. *Anthrozoös, 4,* 226-247.

Baumrind, D. (1973). The development of instrumental competence through socialization. In A. D. Pick (Ed.), *Minnesota Symposium on Child Psychology* (Vol. 7). Minneapolis: University of Minnesota Press.

Bowlby, J. (1969). *Separation and loss.* New York: Basic Books.

Bretherton, I. (1985). Attachment theory: Retrospect and prospect. *Monographs of the Society for Research in Child Development, 50*(109), 3-38.

Bronfenbrenner, U. (1979). *The ecology of human development.* Cambridge, MA: Harvard University Press.

Bronfenbrenner, U. (1986). Ecology of the family as a context for human development. *Developmental Psychology, 22,* 723-742.

Bryant, B. K. (1985). The neighborhood walk: Sources of support in middle childhood. *Monographs of the Society for Research in Child Development, 50*(Issue No. 210).

Bryant, B. K. (1987). *The relevance of pets and neighborhood animals to the social-emotional functioning and development of school-age children.* Final report to the Delta Society, Renton, WA.

Bryant, B. K. (1990). The richness of the child-pet relationships: A consideration of both benefits and cost of pets to children. *Anthrozoös, 3,* 253-261.

Coie, J. D., Dodge, K. A., & Coppotelli, H. (1982). Dimensions and types of social status: A cross age perspective. *Developmental Psychology, 18,* 557-570.

Covert, A. M., Whiren, A. P., Keith, J., & Nelson, C. (1985). Pets, early adolescents and families. *Marriage and Family Review, 8,* 95-108.

Erikson, E. H. (1963). *Childhood and society.* New York: Norton.

Friedmann, E., Katcher, A. H., Thomas, S. A., Lynch, J. J., & Messent, P. R. (1983). Social interaction and blood pressure: The influence of animal companions. *Journal of Nervous and Mental Diseases, 171,* 461-465.

Friedmann, E., Locker, B. Z., & Lockwood, R. (1993). Perception of animals and cardiovascular responses during verbalization with an animal present. *Anthrozoös, 6,* 115-134.

Grotevant, H., & Cooper, C. (1985). Patterns of interaction in family relationships and the development of identity exploration in adolescence. *Child Development, 56,* 415-428.

Kellert, S. R., & Felthous, A. R. (1985). Childhood cruelty toward animals among criminals and noncriminals. *Human Relations, 38,* 1113-1129.

Kidd, A. H., & Kidd, R. M. (1985). Children's attitudes toward their pets. *Psychological Reports, 57,* 15-31.

Kidd, A. H., & Kidd, R. M. (1990a). Factors in children's attitudes toward pets. *Psychological Reports, 66,* 903-910.

Kidd, A. H., & Kidd, R. M. (1990b). Social and environmental influences on children's attitudes toward pets. *Psychological Reports, 67,* 807-818.

Mader, B., Hart, L. A., & Bergin, B. (1989). Social acknowledgments for children with disabilities: Effects of service dogs. *Child Development, 60,* 1263-1277.

McCrindle, C. M. E., & Odendaal, J. S. (1994). Animals in books used for preschool children. *Anthrozoös, 7,* 135-146.

Melson, G. F. (1988). Availability of and involvement with pets by children. *Anthrozoös, 2,* 45-52.

Melson, G. F., Peet, S., & Sparks, C. (1991). Children's attachment to their pets: Links to socio-emotional development. *Children's Environments Quarterly, 8,* 55-65.

Melson, G. F., & Schwarz, R. (1994, October). *Pets as social supports for families with young children.* Paper presented at the annual meeting of the Delta Society, New York.

Melson, G. F., Windecker-Nelson, B., & Schwarz, R. (1997, August). *Support and stress in mothers and fathers of young children.* Paper presented at the annual meeting of the American Psychological Association, Chicago.

Melson, G. F., & Yu, H. (1996). *Caregiving activities of family members.* Unpublished manuscript.

Okagaki, L., & Sternberg, R. J. (1993). Parental beliefs and children's early school performance. *Child Development, 64,* 36-56.

Paul, E. S., & Serpell, J. (1992). Why children keep pets? The influence of child and family characteristics. *Anthrozoös, 5,* 231-244.

Poresky, R. H., & Hendrix, C. (1990). Differential effects of pet presence and pet-bonding on young children. *Psychological Reports, 67,* 51-54.

Rost, D., & Hartmann, A. (1994). Children and their pets. *Anthrozoös, 7,* 242-254.

Rowan, A. (1992). Companion animals demographics and unwanted animals in the United States. *Anthrozoös, 5,* 222-225.

Salmon, P. W., & Salmon, I. (1983). Who owns who? Psychological research into the human-pet bond in Australia. In A. H. Katcher & A. M. Beck (Eds.), *New perspectives on our lives with companion animals* (pp. 244-266). Philadelphia: University of Pennsylvania Press.

Savishinsky, J. (1974). The child is father to the dog: Canines and personality processes in an arctic community. *Human Development, 17,* 460-466.

Shell, M. (1993). *Children of the earth.* New York: Oxford University Press.

Siegler, R. S. (1983). Information-processing approaches to development. In W. Kessen (Ed.), *Handbook of child psychology* (Vol. 1). New York: John Wiley.

Stevenson, H., & Lee, S. (1990). Contexts of achievement. *Monographs of the Society for Research in Child Development, 55*(Issue No. 221).

Stewart, R. B. (1983). Sibling attachment relations: Child-infant interaction in the Strange Situation. *Developmental Psychology, 19,* 192-199.

Wachs, T. E., & Gruen, G. E. (1982). *Early experience and human development.* New York: Plenum.

Waters, E., Vaughn, B. E., Posada, G., & Kondo-Ikemura, K. (1995). Caregiving, cultural, and cognitive perspectives on secure-base behavior and working models. *Monographs of the Society for Research in Child Development, 60*(2-3, Serial No. 244).

Wilson, C. C. (1994). A conceptual framework for human-animal interaction research: The challenge revisited. *Anthrozoös, 7,* 4-12.

Wilson, C. C., & Netting, F. E. (1987). New directions: Challenges for human-animal bond research and the elderly. *Journal of Applied Gerontology, 7,* 51-57.

Impact of Pet Ownership on the Well-Being of Adolescents With Few Familial Resources 15

Nancy M. Bodmer

Abstract

This study focuses on the relationship between pet ownership and well-being of adolescents who report few familial resources. The sample of 752 Swiss adolescents aged between 12 and 16 years (girls and boys were equally represented) contained 405 adolescent pet owners. The impact of pet ownership, demographics (i.e., sex, age, living place, and socioeconomic status), and familial resources (i.e., family climate, daily presence of family members, and amount of leisure time spent with the family) on well-being were evaluated.

Initially, demographic characteristics of pet owners were compared with those of nonowners. Then, the impact of pet ownership on familial resources and on adolescents' well-being was investigated by regression analysis. Pet owners report a higher level of well-being ($p < .05$) and more familial resources ($p < .001$) than nonowners. Neither group of adolescents differ in their socioeconomic status, indicating that a higher living standard does not explain the positive relationships. To detect a moderating effect of pet ownership on the relationship between few familial resources and well-being, a hierarchical regression analysis was run, with no moderating effect shown. Results indicate that pet ownership, although directly related to higher levels of well-being and more familial resources, cannot serve as a buffer for adolescents reporting few familial resources (i.e., the interaction was not significant).

Adolescence is a time of change in many respects and is therefore often viewed as a stormy phase (Erikson, 1968). Recent research has shown that although adolescence involves difficult developmental tasks, in general, stress symptoms are relatively rare. For most adolescents, this time seems to be a harmonious developmental phase (Siddique & D'Arcy, 1984). In addition, adolescents' relationships to their parents and other adults are of a higher quality than has often been assumed. Parental advice is still needed in many areas (Dreher & Dreher, 1985), and family remains an important part of adolescents' lives (Kavsek, 1992). In adolescence, the three basic socializing instances are the family, peers, and school. Of these, family stress has the greatest consequences on the adolescents' well-being (Siddique & D'Arcy, 1984). Girls suffer more than boys under family stress, maybe because they are more socially oriented than boys (Frydenberg & Lewis, 1991).

Positive familial relationships can also be viewed as a protective factor for a successful coping with problems, leading to higher levels of well-being (Bodmer & Grob, 1996; Perrez, 1988; Weber & Laux, 1991). Pets are often treated as part of the family system, fulfilling similar tasks as other family members (Cain, 1979). A relationship with a pet may also serve as a protective factor for an adolescent's well-being. Recent research in several quality of life domains has disclosed the importance of pet ownership for the child's psychosocial and emotional development. Levinson (1980) argued that owning a pet can be related to emotional harmony and stability in humans. Other authors suggest a positive relationship between pet ownership and social well-being (Rost & Hartmann, 1994). It is the unconditional acceptance of a pet that is said to have salutary impact on human health (Sherrick, 1981).

During this century, the European family has been undergoing sociocultural changes. Most obvious of these changes are a relatively high divorce rate and an increased occurrence of new living styles and family types. In the early 1990s, the divorce rate in Switzerland increased to 36%, representing a 1-year increase of 6.6%. In 1992 alone, underage children living with parental divorce increased 10%. The same year, 13.6% of family households were one-parent households (Federal Office for Statistics, 1994). Because of these familial adjustments, all family members experience new constraints. Such circumstances jeopardize the parent-child relationship and indicate that children and adolescents experiencing these stressful familial conditions need an accepting "significant other" to cope with their familial situation. A pet is part of the family system and sometimes the only one who is still available when nobody else is. Families experiencing structural changes are not the only ones living with daily hassles. So-called intact families often experience problems that can lead to family conflicts. In these families, parents might be so stressed that the familial climate is no longer harmonious. Many researchers claim that family processes, especially family conflict, have more serious consequences on adolescents' well-being than the family structure itself (Long, 1986; Partridge & Kotler, 1987). Consequently, family climate and parental involvement in the adolescents' everyday life, rather than family structure, are seen to represent familial resources. Peer influence also increases during adolescence, although the parent-child relationship still remains an important factor of adolescents' well-being. In considering the harmonizing impact of a companion pet on human health, and in arguing that pets are often perceived as a social partner and even as an additional family member, the question arises if pet ownership could be a protective factor for children experiencing few familial resources. Does pet ownership have a positive impact on family climate? Could the availability of a pet at least temporarily replace the emotional nonavailability of a parent? This study seeks answers to these questions by evaluating the relationship between pet ownership and the well-being of adolescents with few or a loss of familial resources.

Method

Participants

This survey was part of the Swiss National Research Program 33, "The Efficacy of Educational Systems." Data presented here were collected in the first wave of a 2-year longitudinal study. In spring 1994, data were obtained from 1,219 German-speaking Swiss students. Those students who had not left school until then were followed and questioned in autumn of the same year. Only those adolescents from the longitudinal sample who answered the question related to possible pet ownership were considered here ($N = 752$). Students were between the ages of 12 to 16 years; girls (49.8%) and boys (50.2%) were equally represented. From the original research program questionnaire, the only variables considered for this survey relate to adolescents' subjective well-being, domains of their family life, and their leisure activities. A more detailed description of the sample and of the instruments used can be found in Grob, Bodmer, and Flammer (1993).

Variables and Procedures

Pet ownership was defined by a positive response to "Have you played with your pet during the last week?" Possible answers were yes or no. Students responding yes were included in the ownership analysis. Demographic variables, categorized by pet owners and nonowners, are described in Table 15.1. Although the question indirectly asked for pet ownership, more important, the question identifies a relationship (this means playing) with the pet.

Other demographic variables evaluated are gender, age, socioeconomic status, living place (i.e., housing type), number of siblings, mother's employment, and family type. Age is dichotomized into two levels (i.e., Level 1 = students aged 12-13; Level 2 = students aged 14-16). To estimate socioeconomic status, the adolescents were asked to indicate if they think that their schoolmates' parents earn as much as, more than, or less than their own parents. The variable living place has three levels. Adolescents were asked to identify whether they live in a house, in a building with less than 10 flats (i.e., apartments), or in a building with 10 flats or more. Further, adolescents were asked for the number of their siblings. This variable is categorized as no sibling, one sibling, two siblings, or three or more siblings. The question related to the mother's employment (working/not working, half-time or less, or more than half-time) indicates the amount of her time spent working outside the home. Finally, adolescents had to indicate with which family members they live permanently. Five family types are of interest for the present study: (1) nuclear family (both biological parents), (2) single-mother family, (3) single-father family, (4) extended family with biological mother and friend or stepfather, and (5) extended family with biological father and friend or stepmother.

The dependent variable, subjective well-being, was drawn from the Bernese Questionnaire on Adolescents' Subjective Well-Being (Grob et al., 1991). This questionnaire consists of six primary and two secondary factors. For this study, two primary factors were selected, "positive attitudes toward life" and "joy in life." These factors were used as an indicator

TABLE 15.1 Comparison of Demographic Variables of Pet and Non-Pet Owners

	Frequencies					
	Owners		*Nonowners*			
	Absolute Frequency	*%*	*Absolute Frequency*	*%*	*Missing*	χ^2
Sex						
Girls	222	55	143	41	—	13.85**; $df = 1$
Boys	183	45	204	59	—	
Age						
Level 5-6	190	47	124	36	—	9.60*; $df = 1$
Level 7-9	215	53	223	64	—	
Socioeconomic status						
Less than	25	7	15	5	47	*ns*
As much as	283	75	251	77	—	
More than	69	18	62	19	—	
Living place					31	19.11**; $df = 2$
House	215	53	132	38	—	
Building (< 10 flats)	123	31	132	38	—	
Building (10 flats or >)	63	16	83	24	—	
Number of siblings						*ns*
None	33	8	35	10	—	
One	211	52	179	52	—	
Two	118	29	89	26	—	
Three or >	43	11	44	13	—	
Employment, mother					17	*ns*
Not employed	160	41	133	39	—	
< 50%	101	25	74	22	—	
Half-time	85	21	80	24	—	
> 50%	51	13	51	15	—	
Family type					110	*ns*
Mother alone	41	10	33	10	—	
Mother & partner	22	5	19	6	—	
Father alone	1	0	4	1	—	
Father & partner	3	1	4	1	—	
Intact family	334	84	181	82	—	

NOTES: $N = 752$; missing values = 92; missing value for the variable family type = 102.
*$p < .01$; **$p < .001$.

for subjective well-being. This new factor, subjective well-being, consists of nine items such as "My future looks good." Cronbach's alpha was relatively high (.81), which corresponds to the published coefficient of the original scale.

Familial resources were operationalized with three components. The first component is a scale of daily activities called "Presence of Family Members." This scale contains 19 questions relating to the presence of family members at different times of the day. Examples are "Are you usually alone for breakfast or is a family member with you?" and "If a family member is with you, who is it?" The second component of the familial resources is another scale of daily activities called "Leisure Activities With Family Members." This scale contains six items, for example, "Do you sometimes go to a restaurant with your family? If yes, how often?" Possible answers are "at least once a week," "once or twice a month," and "more rarely." These two scales were created by the research group and tested in a pilot project with about 300 adolescents.

The third component of the familial resources is the "Family Climate" scale containing two dimensions: "Parent-Child Relationship" and "Conflict Tendency in the Family." The dimension "Parent-Child Relationship" was constructed with five items from the Inventory of Parent and Peer Attachment (Armsden & Greenberg, 1987). These items were translated into German and back into English. The research group added one item to the scale. After the piloting, some of the items had to be slightly adjusted to be better understood by the adolescents. One example item from this scale is "My parents accept me as I am." The dimension "Conflict Tendency in the Family" is represented by three items. For example, questions such as "There are frequent quarrels in our family" are used. This dimension contains two items from the Family Environment Scale (Moos & Moos, 1986). The research group added one item to the scale. Again, the items were slightly adjusted after the piloting. Cronbach's alpha for the "Family Climate" scale, (i.e., two dimensions taken together) was .62. In the following analyses, the two scores of daily activities and the family climate scale taken together will serve as an indicator for "Familial Resources." The reliability of the variable "Familial Resources," the three components taken together, has an unsatisfactory Cronbach's alpha of .51. It is not surprising, however, because the three components measure either qualitative or quantitative aspects and are only partly complementary. To avoid this reliability problem, the indicator "Familial Resources" was used in the analyses only if necessary. Otherwise, the three components were taken separately. This solution allows the differentiation between the importance of the quality and of the quantity of familial resources and also the estimation of the importance of familial resources in general.

Data Analysis

First, possible demographic differences between pet owners and non-owners were analyzed using a chi-square analysis. Variables showing differences were controlled in further analyses to detect a genuine relationship between ownership of a companion animal and adolescents' well-being. Second, both groups of adolescents were compared with respect to their subjective well-being and to their familial resources. Finally, a possible moderating effect of pet ownership on the relationship between familial resources and well-being was analyzed for cases with few familial resources.

Results

First, it was investigated whether pet owners differ from nonowners with respect to their background variables. The results are listed in Table 15.1 (Comparison of Demographic Variables of Pet and Non-Pet Owners). The adolescents of both groups differ significantly for the variables sex, age, and living conditions. More girls than boys own pets. Older pupils (level 7 to 9; ages 14-16) own pets more frequently than younger pupils (level 5 to 6, ages 12-13). Compared with nonowners, pet owners live more frequently in a house rather than in a building. Family structure had no effect on pet ownership. Thus, children and adolescents owning a pet are similarly distributed in the four different family types. Finally, both groups of adolescents do not differ in their own assessment of the socio-economic status of their parents. Thus, pet ownership is no indicator of a higher living standard.

Second, the impact of pet ownership on the adolescents' well-being and on their familial resources was investigated. The first ANOVA was conducted with the factors pet ownership, age, and sex and the dependent variable well-being. Pet ownership shows a significant effect on well-being, F (1, 741) = 5.32, p < .05. Pet owners report higher levels of well-being than nonowners (3.3 > 3.2 on a scale ranging from 1 to 4). Sex and age did not reach the significance level, nor did any of the interactions.

The second ANOVA with the same factors as mentioned above was then conducted on the dependent variable familial resources. The factor pet ownership showed a significant effect, F (1, 744) = 12.62, p < .001. Pet owners show higher values in familial resources than nonowners (5.5 > 5.2 on a scale from 0.5 to 9.5). There was also an age effect, F (1, 744) = 28.92, p < .001, showing that younger adolescents report more familial resources than older adolescents (5.7 > 5.1). The factor sex also reached the significance level, F (1, 744) = 6.27, p < .05. Girls report more resources than boys (5.5 > 5.2). None of the interactions was significant.

To explore the moderating effect of pet ownership on the relationship between familial resources and well-being, a hierarchical regression analysis with demographic variables (sex, age, and living place), pet ownership, and familial resources as predictors was run on the adolescents' well-being (Table 15.2). In the first step, the effect of the Familial Resources × Pet Ownership interaction on the adolescents' well-being was analyzed controlling for the demographic variables and pet ownership. Neither sex nor age nor living place were significant predictors of the adolescents well-being. Pet ownership did not reach the significance level. In a second step, the variables of familial resources (presence of the family, leisure with family, and family climate) as well as the Familial Resources × Pet Ownership interaction were free to enter the equation. Only two predictors showed significant effects on well-being, whereas family climate accounted for 17%; the presence of family members accounted for 1% of the remaining variance. The interaction showed no prediction of well-being. Consequently, the moderator effect of the pet ownership hypothesis could not be confirmed.

Conclusions

Familial bonds, especially the parent-child relationship, are one of the most important protective factors of adolescents' well-being (Siddique & D'Arcy, 1984). Many families suffer from everyday stress due to professional, economic or personal constraints. In Switzerland, the divorce rate is about one third, and many families have to restructure themselves at least one or more times. Such circumstances threaten familial

TABLE 15.2   Hierarchical Analysis Predicting Adolescents' Well-Being

Variables	F	Final β	R^2
Well-being	21.61*		19.05%
Pet ownership		.27	
Demographic variables			
Sex		*ns*	
Age		*ns*	
Living place		*ns*	
Familial resources			
Family climate		.37	17.00%
Family presence		.03	1.00%
Family leisure		.04	
Pet ownership × familial resources		*ns*	

NOTE: $N = 743$; final F-value and βs.
*$p < .001$.

bonds, and the parents may spend less time with their children and become emotionally less available. Family processes, not the family structure, are most relevant for the children's and adolescents' well-being. Often, pets are part of the family, fulfilling similar functions to other family members (Cain, 1979). Pets are always available and offer their affection to everyone needing it. Therefore, owning a pet could have a positive or moderating effect on adolescents' well-being and on their lack of familial resources.

These study data provide support for the hypothesis of a beneficial relationship between pet ownership and adolescents' well-being. Pet owners report higher levels of well-being and more familial resources than nonowners. A significant effect of pet ownership on adolescents' well-being was shown in an analysis of variance. In the regression analysis, pet ownership showed no increase in the explained variance when the demographic variables (sex, age, and living place) were controlled. Girls and older adolescents are more often pet owners. Pet owners also live more frequently in a single-family house rather than in an apartment building. Thus, pet ownership influences positively adolescents' well-being only if these effects are not partialed out. The Pet Ownership × Familial Resources interaction was not significant. This means that in case of few familial resources, pet ownership could barely enhance the relationship between familial resources and well-being.

Further research in this field should seek to demonstrate the positive effects of pet ownership on other areas of the psychosocial well-being of children and adolescents suffering from constraints in different domains. It would be especially interesting to examine longitudinal processes to determine if the loss of familial resources could be mediated by the ownership of a companion animal.

References

Armsden, G. C., & Greenberg, M. T. (1987). The inventory of parent and peer attachment: Individual differences and their relationship to psychological well-being in adolescence. *Journal of Youth and Adolescence, 16,* 427-454.

Bodmer, N. M., & Grob, A. (1996). Bien-être et contraintes desadolescents: Une comparaison entre les adolescents de familles monoparentales et de familles biparentales [Adolescents' well-being and daily hassles: A comparison between adolescents living in one-parent and two-parent families]. *International Journal of Psychology, 31,* 39-48.

Cain, A. (1979). A study of pets in the family system. *Human Behavior, 8,* 24.

Dreher, E., & Dreher, M. (1985). Entwicklungsaufgabe: Theoretisches Konzept und Forschungsprogramm [Developmental task: Theoretical concept and research program]. In R. Oerter (Ed.), *Lebensbewältigung im Jugendalter* [Coping in adolescence] (pp. 30-61). Weinheim, Germany: Edition Psychologie.

Erikson, E. (1968) *Identity, youth and crisis.* New York: Norton.

Federal Office for Statistics. (1994). *Statistical yearbook of Switzerland, 1994.* Zurich, Switzerland: Neue Zürcher Zeitung.

Frydenberg, E., & Lewis, R. (1991). Adolescent coping: The different way in which boys and girls cope. *Journal of Adolescence, 14,* 119-133.

Grob, A., Bodmer, N. M., & Flammer, A. (1993). *Living conditions and the development of adolescents in Europe: The case of Switzerland* (Research Rep. No. 1993-5). Bern, Switzerland: University of Bern, Institute of Psychology.

Grob, A., Lüthi, R., Kaiser, F. G., Flammer, A., Mackinnon, A., & Wearing, A. J. (1991). Berner Fragebogen zum Wohlbefinden Jugendlicher (BFW) [Bernese questionnaire on adolescents' subjective well-being]. *Diagnostica, 37,* 66-75.

Kavsek, M. J. (1992). *Alltagsbewältigung im Jugendalter* [Coping with everyday life in adolescence]. Hamburg, Germany: Kovac.

Levinson, B. M. (1980). The child and his pet: A world of nonverbal communication. In S. A. Corson & E. O. Corson (Eds.), *Ethology and nonverbal communication in mental health* (pp. 111-112). New York: Pergamon.

Long, B. H. (1986). Parental discord versus family structure: Effects of divorce on the self-esteem of daughters. *Journal of Youth and Adolescence, 15,* 19-27.

Moos, R. H., & Moos, B. S. (1986). *Family environment scale.* Palo Alto, CA: Consulting Psychologists Press.

Partridge, S., & Kotler, T. (1987). Self-esteem and adjustment in adolescents from bereaved, divorced, and intact families: Family type versus family environment. *Australian Journal of Psychology, 39,* 223-234.

Perrez, M. (1988). Bewältigung von Alltagsbelastungen und seelische Gesundheit [Coping with daily hassles and mental health]. *Zeitschrift für klinische Psychologie, 4,* 292-306.

Rost, D. H., & Hartmann, A. (1994). Haustierbesitz und sozio-emotionales Wohlbefinden von Kindern [Pet ownership and children's socioemotional well-being]. *Psychologiesche Erziehung und Unterricht, 41,* 241-248.

Sherrick, I. (1981). The significance of pets for children. *Psychoanalytic Study of the Child, 36,* 193-215.

Siddique, C. M., & D'Arcy, C. (1984). Adolescence, stress, and psychological well-being. *Journal of Youth and Adolescence, 13,* 459-473.

Weber, H., & Laux, L. (1991) Bewältigung und Wohlbefinden [Coping and well-being]. In A. Abele & P. Becker (Eds.), *Wohlbefinden: Theorie-Empirie-Diagnostik* (pp. 139-189). Weinheim, Germany: Juventa.

PART VI

The Animal Side of the Coin: Training and Welfare Standards

Dennis C. Turner
Cindy C. Wilson

Up to this point, emphasis has been placed on the role companion animals play in *human* health and quality of life. Relationships and interactions always involve at least two partners, however, and it is imperative that attention be paid to the animal as well. If the animal is improperly selected or trained, or if it is improperly housed such that its welfare is jeopardized, the effectiveness of its service and/or benefits of its companionship will be compromised.

In the first chapter in this section, Duncan addresses the enhanced independence of persons with disabilities after acquiring a service animal and argues that such animals are a valid health care option. The importance of evaluation of the person as a candidate for a service animal, species selection, training standards, and policy are discussed in detail. The person receiving the services, the training program (and trainer), and the animal should all be protected by establishing such standards and policies.

Hubrecht and Turner address the welfare of dogs and cats—the most popular companion animal species—in both private and institutional settings. The general effects of confinement and husbandry practices are discussed, as well as proper housing and matching between people and their animals. Behavioral and physical problems arising from artificial selection and improper housing are also outlined.

The Importance of Training Standards and Policy for Service Animals 16

Susan L. Duncan

Abstract

Service animals promote participation in life's activities, increase independence, and enhance quality of life. A U.S. civil rights law prohibiting discrimination on the basis of disability (Americans With Disabilities Act, 1990) defines *service animal* as any animal that is individually trained to do work or perform tasks for the benefit of a person with a disability. The most common service animals are dogs, although monkeys, cats, and other species have also been reported to serve in this role. Public education and lifestyle support are necessary to optimize the health benefits of the service animal to the individual. This chapter discusses the history, roles, and status of service animals and concludes that the provisional service animal system has not yet provided adequate

AUTHOR'S NOTE: The information contained in this chapter is the result of 4 years of interviews, literature and legislative reviews, participation in forums and symposia, and research and development efforts related to service animal issues. I thank the Delta Society for allowing me access to the information at the National Service Dog Center and Dr. Cindy C. Wilson and Dr. Dennis C. Turner for their support during the preparation of this chapter.

Information on service dogs is available from the National Service Dog Center, Delta Society, 289 Perimeter Road East, Renton, WA 98055-1329; phone (206) 226-7357 ext. 25; TDD (800) 809-2714; fax (206) 235-1076; e-mail NSDC@Compuserve.com.

availability and quality control of trainers and animals, public education, consumer protection, or uniform public health and safety standards. Specific remedies are recommended. A list of suggested topics for further research is available from the author.

Introduction

Animals have been trained to help people with disabilities in the United States for more than 80 years. During this time, the focus of service animal production and supply has been on the training of the animal. There are no uniform standards governing how people become service animal trainers (suppliers), how animals are selected and trained, how individuals are evaluated as candidates to obtain service animals, and whether the animals are matched to an individual's disability-related needs in a therapeutic manner. Similarly, little research has documented the effects of service animals on public health and safety. New applications of service animals and legislation that protects the rights of individuals who have service animals have necessitated greater community interest in all aspects of service animal production and use. Areas of concern are the effects of the animal on the individual who relies on it for help, the effects of the training and the service role on the animal, the implications for training techniques and evaluation by the trainer, and the effects of the service animal on the community.

Disability: Enhancing Independence

Many variables govern the choices a person makes about how to accommodate a disability within his or her lifestyle to promote independence, self-esteem, and productivity. Murray and Lopez (1994) illustrate that different methods used to determine degree of disability can have different outcomes. McDonough, Badley, and Tennant (1995) and Blackford (1993) show that the impact of impairment and disability on an individual is contingent on available resources and social context. Lipstein (1994) succinctly acknowledges the influences of culture and morality on decision making, and Krugman (1994) sums up the influence of advertising on the "likes" and "dislikes" of the contemporary human. Service animals will be the best choice for many people because they enable persons with disabilities to access their environments, increase their autonomy, and participate in activities.

Definition, History, and Roles of Service Animals

Animals providing assistance to persons with disabilities have been referred to by many names, including assistance animals, hearing animals, guide animals, seizure-alert animals, and various "brand names" trademarked by training organizations (e.g., Seeing Eye® dogs). Federal law in the United States (Americans With Disabilities Act, 1990) uses the term *service animal* and defines it as "any animal that is individually trained to do work or perform tasks for the benefit of a person with a disability" (p. 35554).

No one knows when the first service animal was trained. Humanity's historic relationship with the domesticated dog (bred and trained for herding, hunting, protecting, and other types of work) suggests that animals were helping people overcome aspects of disabilities long before the 20th century. Today, the dog is the most common species used in the role of service animal. Although other species, including monkeys, cats, snakes, and birds, have been reported as service animals, there is insufficient documentation of the bioethical and safety considerations of their applications in these roles.

No published studies to date have examined significant populations of trained, healthy, vaccinated service animals for their effects on public health and safety, especially with regard to zoonosis (infection or infectious disease that can be passed from animals to humans) and animal behavior-related risk. Nor have the effects of advanced training, competent handling, and conscientious stewardship (i.e., providing for the animal's care and well-being) on those risks been measured for each species working as service animals. Service dogs, for example, are routinely prohibited from accompanying their owners to Great Britain and other rabies-free areas unless a long quarantine is observed (Bucens & O'Conner, 1990; Fishbein, Corboy, & Saski, 1990; Grandien & Engvall, 1994). Further research can help determine if this policy is too restrictive for a regularly vaccinated, healthy dog that has limited or no opportunity for contact with sources of rabies. Whenever the activity of the animal is restricted, so too is that of the handler.

The primary function of service animals is to address the health care needs of individuals with disabilities, yet scientific and medical literature offers surprisingly little information about the origin, selection, training, and applications of these animals. Standard medical texts (e.g., *Hospital Infections;* Bennett, Brachman, & Sanford, 1992) for the education of health care providers might mention a "seeing eye dog" (p. 312) only in passing. Popular reference materials available to schoolchildren yield somewhat more information: Organized efforts to train service animals began approximately 80 years ago in Germany, when dogs were taught to lead people who had visual impairments (Stuckey, 1982). In the past 30 years, the recognized role of the service animal has expanded. These roles are described in a Delta Society brochure (Duncan, 1995).

- A service animal can alert a person who has hearing impairments to the presence of people and specific sounds.
- A service animal can alert a person who has a seizure disorder to an oncoming seizure. Once alerted, the person can assume a safe position before the seizure begins to avoid injury. The animal will remain with the person through the unconscious phase and help the person reorient when he or she regains consciousness. It is not yet known how an animal can anticipate an oncoming seizure or why it responds behaviorally.
- A service animal can help a person with physical or emotional impairments. It can provide companionship, support, and/or minimal protection; act as a barrier to unwanted physical contact with others or as a social deterrent to criminal victimization; and promote mobility by picking up items, carrying items in a backpack, opening doors, and doing other specific tasks.

Recommending Service Animals as a Health Care Option

A service animal's help can reduce the financial burden of costly equipment, environmental modifications, and human assistance. It can also increase the participation of individuals with disabilities in their activities of daily living and community involvement.

The results of a 2-year study conducted by Allen and Blascovich (1996) document how much less expensive a service dog is than a human care provider. This study involved 48 people with spinal cord injury, muscular dystrophy, multiple sclerosis, and traumatic brain injury. After a service dog is acquired, the cost of paid assistance dropped an average of $13,000 (U.S.) per person per year. The number of hours of paid assistance needed dropped an average of 72%. The participants showed improved self-esteem, independence, community integration, and locus of control. The researchers concluded that these dogs provided health care benefits beyond those of inanimate equipment.

Unlike a human assistant, a service animal is available daily on a 24-hour basis, is portable and versatile, and can do the work of several pieces of assistance equipment. For instance, a person who has limited mobility and uses a walker might instead walk using a cane and a service dog for balance (the dog wears a properly fitted harness that accommodates the person's height and arm position). The benefits could include a more noremalized gait and reduced musculoskeletal side effects from long-term walker use. Even if it cannot replace the walker, the service dog can enable the individual to complete tasks that the dependency on the walker might impede: opening and closing doors and drawers, pulling clothing on and off, retrieving dropped items, standing up after a fall, and carrying groceries.

The growing trend in many countries is to provide rehabilitation efforts that help the person with the disability function effectively in society (Bell, Damrosch, & Lonz, 1994; Brandama, Lakervald, Van Ravensberg, & Heerkens, 1995; Claussen & Nugard, 1994; Friedman, 1993; Harmsen & Noz, 1992; Jackson, Murphy, Dusoir, & Dusoir, 1994; Richardson, 1994; Shakespeare, 1993). Anecdotal reports by many people with service animals indicate that these animals are instrumental in enabling persons to become or remain employed. Maintaining the ability to earn wages can have a positive influence on personal finances as well as on the economy by reducing individuals' need for financial assistance from government sources such as social security disability income, Medicare, and Medicaid.

Choosing service animals can have other advantages for people with disabilities. Additional research documents the general health benefits of companion (pet) animals: reduced blood pressure and increased survival rate following heart attack (Lynch, 1985); improved social contacts (Hart, Hart, & Bergin, 1987; Rossbach & Wilson, 1992; Stallones, 1990; Valentine, Kiddoo, & La Fleur, 1993); improved psychological well-being (Beck & Katcher, 1983; Raveis, Mesagno, Karus, & Gorey, 1993; Zasloff & Kidd, 1994); empathy (Poresky, 1990); facilitated learning and improved communication (Roesenkoetter, 1991); a source of humor (Ackerman, Henry,

Graham, & Coffey, 1994; Herth, 1993); and reduced incidence of minor health problems (Serpell, 1991; Siegel, 1990).

Evaluating a Person as a Candidate for a Service Animal

Although service animals are not suitable for every individual with a disability, they are a health care option that can propel some people toward more functional independence. The success of the person and service animal as a team is affected by factors such as these:

- Thorough evaluation of the person's needs
- Ability of the animal to be trained to reliably meet the individual's needs
- Ability of the person to provide for the stewardship of the animal
- Availability of adequate training for both the person and the animal
- Acceptance and support of the person and service animal from the family, health care and social service providers, and the community,

People with disabilities associated with many diagnoses can benefit from service animals. Appraisal of a person as a candidate for a service animal should include consideration of the person's ability to function on a daily basis. Haley, Coster, and Binda-Sundberg (1994) describe the importance of considering context when clinically interpreting the significance of a person's disability. Before recommending a service animal, the health care professional should assemble a client profile that identifies and evaluates the following client characteristics:

- Difficulties with activities of daily living: A service animal can ensure task completion and make activities accessible. An evaluation of ergonomic requirements should be included in this assessment to ensure that the individual can easily interact with the animal and related equipment without compromising his or her health status.
- Stamina: The person conserves energy when the animal performs tasks. The fatigue-inducing effects of stress, related to repeated attempts to perform a task completely and the apprehension felt when facing a difficult task, can be mitigated by a service animal.
- Level of activity: A service animal can help the person get more exercise and be more mobile. Providing care, exercise, and grooming affords opportunities

for physical activity. Specific human-animal interactive regimens can be designed and incorporated into physical, occupational, and recreational therapy planning.

- Level of social integration: An animal can be a distraction from the disability and facilitate interaction with others. Previously cited studies by Allen and Blascovich (1996), Hart et al. (1987), Rossbach and Wilson (1992), Stallones (1990), and Valentine et al. (1993) have shown that the presence of an animal makes a person appear more approachable.

- Focus of attention: An animal can help the person externalize his or her attention and provide motivation for activities that promote wellness. Feelings of being needed and sharing experiences with another living being can be powerful motivators for taking care of one's self.

- Safety factors: The animal's presence can alleviate some of the safety and well-being concerns of the individual and of friends and family who cannot be with the person all day. This can reduce some of the stress that occurs in interpersonal relationships when significant others must also assume the roles of caregivers.

- Nutritional status: The animal can improve the person's access to food by opening the food storage area or carrying food to the person or because the person synchronizes his or her meals with the animal's.

- Ability to work: The animal can provide the physical or emotional support necessary to help the person stay employed.

- Support systems: Adequate financial and community support will enhance the benefits of the service animal. This includes follow-up training for dog and handler if necessary, access to public areas (including housing, employment, and transportation), provision for care and feeding of animal and individual, and an atmosphere of social acceptance.

- Cognitive ability: The handler must be able to provide for the behavioral management and stewardship of the animal.

Species Selection and Animal Welfare

Equally important considerations are those that determine the appropriate animal to be trained to meet the individual's needs (Kaufmann, 1996). The impact that the training process and role expectations have on the well-being of the animal and the ability of the individual to provide for the animal's well-being are critical to protecting the welfare of the animal. People with service animals are not necessarily exempt from animal control and welfare laws, including leash, breed or species restrictions, and cruelty regulations. An animal's welfare can be severely jeopardized when it is poorly maintained or managed or subjected to performance or lifestyle expectations that are detrimental for that animal. An unhealthy, poorly behaved, stressed, or otherwise inappropriate service animal can be hazardous to the individual and the community.

Training and Distribution of Service Animals

The production and assignment of service animals have been primarily the realm of animal trainers; people who want service animals contact trainers for guidance and assistance. Although the public generally believes that service animals are uniformly trained and evaluated, there are no uniform standards for the training or evaluation of all service animals. Nor are there uniform expertise requirements or standards for the animal trainers. There has never been developed a widely available body of knowledge based on credible research for the education of trainers, the training of dogs, or the education of handlers. People who train service dogs either develop their own techniques or apprentice to learn another trainer's methods. In most states, only a business license is required to train service dogs for others. This applies as much to the training of dogs that do guide work as it does to the training of dogs for other purposes. Although some trainer fraternal organizations suggest guidelines for members, those guidelines are not enforceable for nonmembers and do not prevent noncompliant members from legally being able to continue to train animals.

Without the benefit of a validated preparatory education or consistent opportunities for professional development, service animal trainers have had to interpret consumer health care and other relevant data (social service, financial, and lifestyle) to train and supply service animals. The burden has been on the trainer to assess the consumer's immediate medical needs, lifestyle, and prognosis throughout the estimated working life span of the animal. The responsibilities of a service animal trainer include the following:

- Selection of an animal that can be trained to reliably perform the desired work for the consumer without posing a threat to public health and safety
- Assessment of the handler's disability-related needs
- Assessment of the handler's abilities to manage the animal's behavior

- Determination of a training process that is humane, well suited to the animal's method of learning, and successfully transferable to the handler
- Assessment of the handler's lifestyle and the positive and negative impacts of that lifestyle on the service animal
- Evaluation of the ability of the handler to provide for the stewardship of the animal
- Determination of the need for follow-up training of the animal and/or education of the handler

Other global issues that must be considered by the trainer include ethical business practices such as maintenance of confidentiality of handler data, pricing practices, legal ownership of the animal, achievable guarantees of product quality, and familiarity with current laws that protect service animals, their handlers, and public health and safety.

The abilities of trainers to address these considerations and the quality of the service animals they supply vary widely. Because there have never been uniform requirements for all trainers to meet standards of professional expertise, trainers in business today might have been training service animals very well for 20 years or very poorly for 20 years or might have just begun producing service animals. Yet they are still expected to produce high-quality service animals for people with increasingly sophisticated disability-related needs.

Acquiring a Trained Service Animal

People with disabilities who wish to acquire a service animal often find that obtaining trained service animals is difficult and time-consuming. Some people do not even know that service animals are an option. Of the estimated 54 million Americans with disabilities, a mere 16,000 individuals—less than 0.03%—are estimated to have service dogs, and half of those are believed to be dogs that do only guide work. This discrepancy is affected by several factors. The lack of a formal education system for trainers reduces the number of competent service animal trainers and limits the availability of service animals. Health care providers are not routinely educated about the roles and applications of service animals or how to evaluate clients for candidacy. Thus the recommendation rate is low. Public education about service animals is sporadic and often contains inaccurate and incomplete information about the range of service animal work, legitimate uses of service animals as disability-related medical interventions, and the laws that protect individuals with disabilities who have service animals in public places. This inhibits an individual's ability to easily locate a reliable source of service animal information or to function optimally with a trained service animal.

To obtain a trained service animal, a person must meet the arbitrary candidacy criteria of the service animal supplier. This may prevent a significant portion of people with disabilities who could benefit from a service animal from acquiring one.

The cost of the service animals varies by supplier. Service dogs, for example, can range from no cost to $20,000 or more. At this time, no third-party payer consistently reimburses for the costs of service animal acquisition and maintenance. To pay for a service animal, the person with the disability might be forced to seek fund-raising efforts on his/her behalf from community organizations.

The consumer must typically wait from several months to many years for a service animal to be available and might have to travel long distances and stay at a training site for extended periods to obtain the animal and complete handler training. Individuals who want a service animal in a more time- and cost-effective manner and who are capable of training their own animals have great difficulty locating information about the appropriate selection and training of service animals.

Information requests made to the Delta Society National Service Dog Center in 1995 and 1996 show that concerns are being voiced about the service dog provisional system. These concerns come from several sources.

Trainers want
- A reliable, validated mechanism to guide the selection and training of service animals
- A system for professional development

People with disabilities want
- Adequate information so they can be prepared consumers when selecting a service animal source
- A method to determine if service animal suppliers are legitimate
- Readily available resources for trained service animals
- Quality control measures to ensure that their service animals are healthy, well behaved, and well trained to meet individual needs

- Consistent, legally protected support to function optimally within their own communities and in the communities that they visit

Health care providers want
- Comprehensive information about how service animals can help clients with disabilities
- Assistance for consumers with service animal-associated costs
- Assurances that service animals and training assistance will be available as needed for their clients

Animal welfare organizations want
- Assurances that service animals are humanely trained and handled and well suited for the type of work they are trained for, in the environments in which they are expected to perform

Public accommodations and the general public want
- Assurances that animals presented in public are genuine service animals and present no risk to public health and safety

Perspective, Participation, Progress

Historically, the process of producing trained service animals has been a charity-motivated endeavor applied to a limited population within a population minority. The increase in the number of people with disabilities who could benefit from service animals, along with the recent changes in legislation that protect people with disabilities who have service animals, has helped redefine the field of service animal provision not merely as an animal training or philanthropic effort but as a health care and public policy matter as well.

For service animals to be viable choices to help individuals overcome the limitations of disabilities, health care providers, trainers, handlers, policymakers, and communities must work together to support the handler-service dog team. This can be achieved by the development of the following.

An accessible, validated, humane, and comprehensive system for people to learn to become competent service animal trainers. This system should be multidisciplinary (including input from experts on training, animal behavior and welfare, public health and safety, health care and social service providers, educators, and others) and predicated on scientific principles regarding the way animals and people learn. Standardized language is needed to improve communications between participants. Provision of advanced and specialty continuing education programs would provide professional credibility, acknowledge the trainer's level of achievement, and provide for professional growth.

A validated accreditation system for trainers, administered by an independent organization that is not directly involved in the training of service animals. Applied equally to each trainer and animal, this would provide objectively measured quality control standards to help identify capable service animal suppliers and trained animals that meet measurable levels of quality. This system can be voluntary or mandatory and connected to business or state licensure requirements for trainers. Accreditation can require proof of professional development (attendance of classes designated for continuing education credit, skills evaluations by accrediting body, etc.) and can be awarded in multiple levels, from basic to advanced or specialized. Accreditation by itself will not eliminate incompetent or unethical trainers as suppliers but will serve as an indicator of professional expertise.

State licensure to practice as a trainer, based on completion of competency testing, with consistent requirements for licensure in all geographic areas. In addition to registering trainers who meet minimum capability criteria, this would help eliminate incompetent or unethical trainers through license revocation if the trainer failed to meet minimum criteria in practice (on the basis of failure of licensing test or complaints). Provisions can be made to track license applicants to ensure that a trainer whose license was revoked in one area cannot obtain a second license in another. Licensing and accreditation systems should be carefully evaluated for their pros and cons. Some argue that there is already too much governmental regulation and that voluntary accreditation alone is adequate, as it is for the American Association of Zoos and Aquaria or the American Association of Laboratory Animal Care. The main difference is that the service animal trainer directly ministers to the needs of individuals with disabilities. Practitioners in other health care-affiliated fields who provide direct intervention must assume a high level of professional responsibility through licensure. Trainers have access to a consumer's confidential health (and possibly financial) data, have repeated contact with the consumer (sometimes in the consumer's home) and might have physical contact during training. Having a medical condition that substantially limits one or more major life activities places individuals with disabilities in a higher risk category for injury and victimization (Tobin, 1992). The consumer is entitled to enforceable guarantees of confidentiality, safety, and reassurance that his or her health status will not be compromised by well-intentioned but ill-advised interactions with the trainer or service animal.

Well-defined regulations governing trainer liability. The regulations should provide answers to questions such as this: What are the trainer's responsibilities if the animal does not perform tasks as expected or if training methods have an adverse affect on the animal's disposition or behavior?

Clear training and handling guidelines regarding humane techniques and maintenance of animal welfare. Species well suited for service work should be identified. A centralized registration system for service animals could help identify trends in service animal production (species/breeds, numbers, type of work done, etc.) and could be used to help reassign trained service animals to new owners if their original owners no longer desired or were unable to care for the animals.

Consistent public policies that use the same terminology and definitions. These policies should provide the same protections to individuals with service dogs in public places regardless of geopolitical boundaries. These policies will enhance individuals' abilities to maintain functional independence through better access to goods and services at public accommodations. Policies should be based on research that measures the actual risks of healthy, well-trained service animals in those public places. A person with a service animal should be able to secure housing, maintain employment, use public transportation, go to school, have a meal at a restaurant, and participate in other common activities without having to meet separate criteria at each place to "prove" that the service animal is legitimate. National and international cooperation will expedite this process.

A body of credible research relevant to service animal production and application. Only a small amount of published research exists that is specific to service animals, although anecdotal reporting accrues in greater amounts each year. Strategic, validated studies will contribute to the theoretical basis of service animal selection, training and application, and public policy development.

Systems to provide financial assistance for service animal costs. Reimbursement for acquisition and maintenance costs of service animals could be offered by third-party payers on schedules similar to those established for other durable medical equipment. Reimbursement is not yet a routine benefit of health care plans. This type of guaranteed funding would help stimulate greater interest in service animal training as a career option and help consumers obtain service animals as a recommended health care option in the same category as eyeglasses, a cane, or a wheelchair.

Comprehensive and consistent education about service animals, made available especially to health care and social service providers, policymakers, public entity employees, and people with disabilities. This can be achieved through inclusion in basic professional education, employee orientation, and continuing education programs.

The training and application of a service animal involves much more than teaching Spot the dog to sit. Research such as that by Allen and Blascovich (1996) and supportive legislation for people who have service animals corroborate the idea of service animal production and maintenance as a multidisciplinary issue. Health care, human rights, consumer protection, animal welfare and training, and public health and safety are all important components. These broad implications offer each member of the community the opportunity to contribute his or her expertise and to participate in the process that will improve the quality of life for individuals who rely on service animals. Thorough education about service animals will prepare each discipline for its role. Health care providers can assess the specific health needs of the individual, recommend service animals for those who are appropriate candidates, and evaluate the effects of the service animal on the person. Trainers can learn to effectively train animals, educate handlers, and communicate with providers as part of the health care team. People with disabilities can be informed consumers and make intelligent choices about service animals. Policymakers can make reasonable and fair policies that consistently protect the individual's right to function with a service dog in public places. The general public can recognize and support the efforts of the individual to achieve greater independence and dignity with the help of a reliable, well-behaved service animal.

References

Ackerman, M. H., Henry, M. B., Graham, K. M., & Coffey, N. (1994). Humor won, humor too: A model to incorporate humor into the healthcare setting. *Nursing Forum, 29*(2), 15-21.

Allen, K., & Blascovich, J. (1996). The value of service dogs for people with severe ambulatory disabilities. *Journal of the American Medical Association, 275*(13), 1001-1006.

Americans With Disabilities Act of 1990, 42 U.S.C. § 12101 et seq.

Beck, A., & Katcher, A. (1983). *Between pets and people: The importance of animal companionship.* New York: G. P. Putnam.

Bell, R. W., Damrosch, S. P., & Lonz, E. R. (1994). The polio survivor as expert: Implications for rehabilitation nursing research. *Rehabilitation Nursing, 19*(4), 198-202, 258.

Bennett, J. V., Brachman, P. S., & Sanford, J. P. (1992). Basic consideration of hospital infections: Inanimate environment: Animal visitation. In J. V. Bennett, P. S. Brachman, & J. P. Sanford (Eds.), *Hospital infections (3rd ed., pp. 312-313). Boston: Little, Brown.*

Blackford, K. A. (1993). Erasing mothers with disabilities through Canadian family-related policy. In Citizens of the state? The experience of disabled people [Special issue]. *Disability, Handicap and Society, 8*(3), 281-294.

Brandama, J. W., Lakervald, H. K., Van Ravensberg, D. D., & Heerkens, Y. F. (1995). Reflection on the definition of impairment and disability as defined by the World Health Organization. *Disability and Rehabilitation, 17*(3-4), 119-127.

Bucens, M., & O'Conner, L., (1990). Rabies and the traveller. *Australian Family Physician, 19*(2), 157-161.

Claussen, B., & Nugard, J. F. (1994). Patients who are in danger of being dropped from the labour-market [On-line]. *Tidsskrift For Den Norske Laegeforenins, 114*(16), 1811-1814. Abstract from: MedLine Item 94350375

Duncan, S. L. (1995). *Healthcare options: Service animals for people who have disabilities* [Brochure]. Renton, WA: Delta Society.

Fishbein, D. B., Corboy, J. M., & Saski, D. M. (1990). Rabies prevention in Hawaii. *Hawaii Medical Journal, 49*(3), 98-101.

Friedman, S. (1993). Accommodation issues in the work place for people with disabilities: A needs assessment in an educational setting. *Disability, Handicap and Society, 8*(1), 3-23.

Grandien, M., & Engvall, A. (1994). Quarantine to be abolished for animals and cats: New regulations for import of pets from EU/EFTA countries [On-line]. *Lakartidningen, 91*(5), 373-374. Abstract from: MedLine Item 94158413

Haley, S. M., Coster, W. J., & Binda-Sundberg, K. (1994). Measuring physical disablement: The contextual challenge. *Physical Therapy, 74*(5), 443-451.

Harmsen, A. J., & Noz, M. (1992). Promoting work during the sick leave period through cooperation between health insurance physician and the attending physician [On-line]. *Nederlands Tijdschrift Voor Geneeskunde, 135*(39), 1920-1922. Available: MedLine Item 93025155)

Hart, L., Hart, B., & Bergin, B. (1987). Socializing effects of service animals for people with disabilities. *Anthrozoös, 1*(1), 41-44.

Herth, K. A. (1993). Humor and the older adult. *Applied Nursing Research, 6*(4), 146-153.

Jackson, A. J., Murphy, P. J., Dusoir, T., & Dusoir, H. (1994). Ophthalmic, health and social profile of guide animal owners in Northern Ireland. *Ophthalmic and Physiological Optics, 14*(4), 371-377.

Kaufmann, M. (1996). The controversy over exotic service animals. *Alert, 7,* 3.

Krugman, H. E. (1994). Pavlov's animal and the future of consumer psychology. *Journal of Advertising Research, 34*(6), 67.

Lipstein, O. J. (Ed.). (1994, March-April). Culture and morality: Is it wrong to eat your animal? *Psychology Today, 27*(2), 15.

Lynch, J. (1985). *The language of the heart.* New York: Basic Books.

McDonough, P. A., Badley, E. M., & Tennant, A. (1995). Disability, resources, role demands and mobility handicap. *Disability and Rehabilitation, 17*(3-4), 159-168.

Murray, D. J., & Lopez, A. D. (1994). Quantifying disability: Data, methods and results. *Bulletin of the World Health Organization, 72*(3), 481-494.

Poresky, R. H. (1990). The young children's empathy measure: Reliability, validity and effects of companion animal bonding. *Psychological Reports, 65*(5), 931-936.

Raveis, V. H., Mesagno, F., Karus, D., & Gorey, E. (1993). *Pet ownership as a protective factor supporting the emotional well-being of cancer patients and their family members.* New York: Memorial Sloan-Kettering Cancer Center, Department of Social Work Research Unit.

Richardson, M. (1994). The impact of the Americans With Disabilities Act on employment opportunity for people with disabilities. *Annual Review of Public Health, 15,* 91-105.

Roesenkoetter, M. M. (1991). Health promotion: The influence of pets on life patterns in the home. *Holistic Nursing Practice, 5*(2), 42-51.

Rossbach, K. A., & Wilson, J. P. (1992). Does an animal's presence make a person appear more likable? *Anthrozoös, 5*(1), 40-51.

Serpell, J. (1991). Beneficial effects of pet ownership on some aspects of human health and behavior. *Journal of the Royal Society of Medicine, 84*(12), 717-720.

Siegel, J. M. (1990). Stressful life events and use of physician services among the elderly: The moderating role of pet ownership. *Journal of Personality and Social Psychology, 58*(6), 1081-1086.

Shakespeare, T. (1993). Disabled people's self-organization: A new social movement? In Citizens of the state? The experience of disabled people [Special issue]. *Disability, Handicap and Society, 8*(3), 249-264.

Stallones, L. (1990, Fall). Companion animals and health of the elderly. *People, Animals and Environment,* 18-19.

Stuckey, K. (Ed.). (1982). *The world book encyclopedia* (Vol. 8). Chicago: World Book-Childcraft International.

Tobin, P. (1992, December). Addressing special vulnerabilities in prevention. *National Resource Center on Child Sexual Abuse News, 5,* 14.

Valentine, D. P., Kiddoo, M., & La Fleur, B. (1993). Psychosocial implications of service animal ownership for people who have mobility or hearing impairments. *Social Work in Health Care, 19*(1), 109-125.

Zasloff, R. L., & Kidd, A. H. (1994). Loneliness and pet ownership among single women. *Psychological Reports, 74,* 747-752.

Companion Animal Welfare in Private and Institutional Settings 17

Robert Hubrecht
Dennis C. Turner

Abstract

This chapter explores dog and cat welfare in private and institutional settings. Aspects of cruelty and neglect, confinement, behavior problems, physical problems resulting from artificial selection (and manipulative operations on dogs), and owner-animal matching are discussed for both companion animal species in home settings. Four aspects of dog kennel design considered are social housing, space and structure, visibility, and noise levels. Welfare aspects of cats in shelters and asylums, in breeding catteries, at cat exhibitions, and in animal-assisted activity or therapy programs are explored. For both species, the latest research data serve as the basis for discussion and recommendations. Because the responsibilities and capabilities for ensuring optimum dog and cat welfare are most often in human hands, private and institutional owners have a moral and, in some cases, legal obligation to do so. Interactions and relationships with cats and dogs must be based on principles of responsible ownership and trusteeship.

Past conferences on human-animal interactions have always placed primary emphasis on the human partner and the potential benefits from interaction with companion animals (Anderson, Hart, & Hart, 1984; Fogle, 1981; Katcher & Beck, 1983; IEMT, 1985;

Rowan, 1988). The Geneva Conference on "Animals, Health, and Quality of Life" in 1995 was no different, although the organizers attempted to attract more contributions from animal behavior and welfare specialists (personal observation). The human-animal relationship is indeed a partnership involving two parties, and it behooves us to consider it from the animal's point of view and its quality of life, not just that of the person involved (Turner, 1984, 1991a, 1991b, 1995a, 1995b; Turner & Stammbach-Geering, 1990). If the animal is not properly housed and cared for in a private or institutional setting, or if it is stressed during animal-assisted activities, it is probable that the human-animal relationship will not develop harmoniously, jeopardizing the animal's welfare and any potential therapeutic benefit from the relationship (Turner, 1992, 1995c, 1996a). Because dogs and cats are most often involved in therapeutic programs, this chapter reviews selected aspects of dog and cat welfare.

The Dog and Its Welfare

Most dog owners consider themselves able to judge whether their dogs are happy or not. Despite the large body of research on the dog, however, it is not a simple matter to prove whether a dog is stressed or whether its housing and husbandry are adequate. Much information is known about the dog and its physiology (Blythe, Gannon, & Craig, 1994; MacArthur, 1987). Yet despite this knowledge and the length of time that the dog has lived with humans as a domestic pet—more than 14,000 years (Clutton-Brock, 1995)—surprisingly little is known about the dog's behavioral needs and requirements.

Animals have adapted to behave in different ways from humans. In addition, their senses and perceptions are different. Although it is possible to identify the limits of their senses, animals' experience of the world is something at which humans can only guess. Nevertheless, sensible judgments can be made on the welfare impacts of different housing systems for dogs, which include institutions such as rescue shelters, quarantine kennels, purpose-built kennels for working or service dogs, and laboratory housing, as well as the home environment.

One approach (Webster, 1994) to assessing the welfare of animals in various situations is to test the proposed housing system against the five freedoms as revised by the United Kingdom Farm Animal Welfare Council

(FAWC; 1993). These state that animals should be housed in conditions with

1. Freedom from thirst, hunger and malnutrition—by ready access to fresh water and a diet to maintain full health and vigor
2. Freedom from discomfort—by providing an appropriate environment including shelter and a comfortable resting area
3. Freedom from pain, injury or disease—by prevention or rapid diagnosis and treatment
4. Freedom to express normal behavior—by providing sufficient space, proper facilities and company of the animal's own kind
5. Freedom from fear and distress—by ensuring conditions which avoid mental suffering (pp. 3-4)

Freedoms 1, 2, and 3 can easily be provided by good husbandry and veterinary care. Most pet keepers and professionals dealing with dogs are able to make a fairly accurate judgment on whether a dog is suffering as a consequence of a violation of one of these freedoms. Unfortunately, it is not as easy to arrive at a consensus on what normal behaviors the dog should have freedom to express. Likewise, some owners may also lack a sufficient knowledge of dogs and their biology to accurately judge whether their dogs are undergoing mental suffering.

Dog Welfare in the Home

Generally speaking, the dog is well adapted for living closely with humans. If puppies (between the ages of 3 and 13 weeks) are given appropriate opportunities for socialization with dogs and humans, they subsequently have the ability to bond with both humans and other dogs. The dog is also relatively easy to train using appropriate techniques so that it can be used for a variety of purposes, such as guarding, hunting, or assistance. The dog as a pet has evolved from the dog as a working animal (Coppinger & Schneider, 1995). Both conscious and unconscious artificial selection has changed the physical and behavioral characteristics of dogs from those of their ancestral wolf. A review of the changes is provided by Bradshaw and Brown (1990). The dog's success as a companion animal is partly due to the fortuitous match of its natural social system with that imposed on it in the human-dog relationship (preadaptation) and partly a result of human selection for desired characteristics.

In affluent nations, a dog's welfare in the home is likely to be substantially greater than it could expect in the wild or under feral conditions. In most cases, the dog is provided with shelter, warmth, food, and veterinary attention when appropriate. Moreover, the domestic dog is provided with a social life that mimics some of the features of that of a pack. This, together with opportunities for socializing with other dogs either in the same home or while being exercised, can provide a rich and stimulating environment.

Cruelty and Neglect

Domestic conditions vary widely, and there are cases in which dog suffering occurs as a result of either deliberate or unconscious cruelty. Many such cases are due to neglect (Hubrecht, 1995b), which may result from ignorance or a lack of appreciation of the long-term responsibilities of pet ownership. It is fortunate that the more obviously deliberate cases of cruelty are relatively rare, but dogs may suffer just as much whether or not the cruelty is intentional. Dogs may stray through either accident or neglect. Such strays, apart from representing a nuisance and hazard to humans, may suffer from disease or accident and are unlikely to receive adequate care (Hubrecht, 1995b). The activities of the various welfare shelters and rescue organizations are extremely valuable in coping with this problem, and many of them provide education programs for humans and neutering programs for the dogs, both of which help reduce the incidence of strays.

Confinement

Domestication inevitably involves some confinement. Thus, there is the potential for suffering if the conditions do not meet the needs of the dog. Excessive confinement in a small enclosure or tethering for long periods can certainly be cruel, although it does seem that exercise itself might not be as important as previously thought (Clark, Calpin, & Armstrong, 1991). The problems arising from confinement from the animal's point of view are likely to result from (a) the restriction on its ability to perform normal behavior, (b) the restraint itself, and/or (c) the dog's inability to maintain social contact with humans or other dogs (Hubrecht, Serpell, & Poole, 1992). The animal's difficulties in coping with these conditions may be shown by various behavioral abnormalities that can include locomotory stereotypes or excessive barking. Restricted environments early in life can have a destructive effect on the dog's later character (Hubrecht, 1995b; Serpell & Jagoe, 1995). Fearful and phobic behavior, a common outcome, is clearly detrimental to the animal's welfare and also results in a poor-quality pet. It is becoming more common in the Western world for both partners to work, and leaving the dog alone at home may lead to separation-related problems. Such problems suggest that the dog is undergoing some anxiety and probably experiencing a strong motivation to regain contact with its owners. Again, experiences during the animal's development are likely to be important in determining whether a susceptible animal develops such behaviors (Serpell & Jagoe, 1995).

Behavior Problems

Aggression is one of the least acceptable and one of the most common canine behavior problems (Hart & Hart, 1985, cited in Serpell & Jagoe, 1995) and may be the product of different stimuli. Serpell and Jagoe review the development of these and other problems and show that certain early events in the dog's life can have an influence on the dog's likelihood of showing behavioral problems later in life. Unresolved behavior problems can lead to the abandonment, euthanasia, or maltreatment of dogs. It is therefore vital that the general public and veterinarians should be aware that many such problems can be overcome by appropriate training, handling, or other therapies.

Physical Problems

Artificial Selection

Artificial selection has produced a well-domesticated animal, but it has also led to some of the widest variation in physical form seen in one species. The precise way in which these variations have arisen remains unclear (Coppinger & Schneider, 1995). Owners have selected for desired physical forms in pedigree animals, but some features may have arisen as a by-product of selection for other traits. Whatever the etiology, the various dog breeds suffer from more than 400 inherited diseases (Sargan, 1995). In most cases, it is clear that the welfare of dogs with these deformities is impaired, and it is incumbent on breeders not to select for extreme forms and to avoid breeding from animals that develop problems.

Docking and Cropping

Cropping dogs' ears and docking their tails are long-standing practices that are now controversial. These procedures are usually carried out soon after birth, and the protagonists for these practices argue that they seem to cause little pain, that they improve the appearance of the dog, and that docking tails reduces injuries to the tails of hunting dogs searching through thorny undergrowth. Cropping ears is illegal in the United Kingdom, but tail docking is still carried out by veterinary surgeons, although supposedly only for "therapeutic or acceptable prophylactic reasons." Docking is usually carried out without anesthetic. Because the puppy's peripheral nervous system is functioning, docking must cause pain, although there is little information about the puppy's perception of the pain. The lack of an apparently large pain response may be due to poor observation of subtle indications or may possibly be because the puppy's motor responses are not fully developed. Two major studies have been carried out on injury rates of docked and undocked breeds. Although both studies suffered from flaws (Bonner, 1995), it is interesting that the injury rates to tails or tail stumps reported in an Edinburgh study were 0.41% for undocked dogs and 0.31% for docked dogs. These extremely low rates of injury are certainly less than the injury caused by docking itself. Any nonessential mutilation of an animal is undesirable and reduces the animal's welfare.

Owner-Dog Matching

Every day, animal shelters provide a service similar to that of a dating agency. A rehomed dog should be well matched with its new owner; it is then much less likely to be returned to the shelter, and both dog and owner will enjoy a better quality of life. Unfortunately, until recently there has been little research into methods of effectively matching the temperaments of dogs and owners. It is known that breed-specific differences in behavior (Bradshaw, Goodwin, Lea, & Whitehead, 1996; Willis, 1995) and hence behavioral needs can be extremely important, but there have been few behavioral studies of these differences. Another problem is that the difficulty of assessing the potential owner can be as great as that of assessing the dog. Hence, breed variation, individual differences in both dogs and humans, and differences in the various circumstances of households all provide the potential for dog-owner mismatches which may lead to the dog's suffering.

A number of animal rescue organizations have developed their own methods of testing the character of dogs, but these are usually invalidated. Dog assessment tests normally involve placing the dog in a number of situations such as play and introducing the dog to another, mild stimuli such as ringing bells or dropped keys (Ledger, Baxter, & McNicholas, 1995; Wickens et al., 1995). Through the use of an intelligent and flexible approach, it should be possible to identify some features of the dog's character, to decide what sort of home the dog would be best adapted to, and to identify selected behavioral problems.

Dogs in Institutions

Not all dogs spend their entire lives in a domestic environment. In many cases, they may be housed in various types of institutions for at least a part of their lives. Examples include quarantine kennels, boarding kennels, kennels for greyhound racing, training establishments for assistance animals such as guide dogs or hearing dogs, hunting kennels, and kennels for dogs used by the police and the armed forces. Dogs are also used in the experimental development of some pharmaceuticals and in regulatory toxicology studies. The welfare of these animals clearly depends not only on the quality of the kennels but also on the purpose for which they are kept.

A number of organizations produce assistance dogs for people with various disabilities. These dogs usually have to undergo a period in kennels during training, and this, together with the training itself, may be stressful for some dogs (Vincent, 1993). The best-known assistance dogs are those for people with sensory disabilities, such as guide dogs and hearing dogs, but the different uses to which dogs are put has been growing. Some assistance dogs are used as physical supports by disabled persons when maneuvering into or out of their chairs. Depending on the conformation of the dog and the weight of the disabled person, there may be some risk of damage to the dog's back. Other activities can also place undue stresses on the dog's frame. A recent booklet has been published (Coppinger, 1995) on the mechanical forces to which wheelchair assistance dogs are subjected while carrying out tasks such as opening doors or pulling a wheelchair. The booklet shows how poor harness design can lead to excessive and poorly balanced loads on the dog and provides excellent advice on how to improve the various harness systems.

The Dog and Kennel Design: Conflicting Requirements?

Kennels should be designed to meet the dog's needs to the greatest extent compatible with the function of the kennel and the needs of care-giver. The dog's needs are likely to vary, depending on breed, duration of stay, and proportion of the day that the dog is expected to remain within the kennel. Generally, much current dog housing has been designed primarily to confine the dog in a state of good physical health and to meet the requirements of the users. These are, of course, important functions, but the mental requirements of the dog are usually unnecessarily neglected. Recommendations for kennel design improvements have been developed that take canine behavior into account and are based on research and a review of the available literature (Hubrecht, 1993b).

Social Housing

In kennels that house large numbers of dogs, the pressures on staff are often such that contact time with the dogs becomes limited (Hubrecht et al., 1992). A good kennel design should be flexible enough to house the dogs socially in harmonious groups where possible and also to allow separation of animals where necessary. Single housing for prolonged periods is likely to be deleterious to the dog and is associated with an increased incidence of behavioral abnormalities (Hetts, 1991). Single housing may sometimes be necessary, however, for health purposes or because of aggression. There are no data to indicate what an optimum group size might be, but pair housing seems to be a reasonable compromise; dogs in pairs spend a similar proportion of their time socializing to that in larger groups (Hubrecht, 1993a). Aggression in group housing can be a serious problem, in some cases leading to the death of animals. Thus, it is important to ensure an adequate husbandry routine to monitor the dogs and prevent potential problems.

Space and Kennel Structures

Whatever the group size, the pen must provide adequate space for the dogs to walk for at least a few paces in a straight line. Small pens limit normal behavior expression and are associated with a higher prevalence of circling and other stereotypes (Hubrecht et al., 1992). Larger pens with separate sleeping and exercise areas provide a more complex and interesting environment and permit social housing. Larger pens also allow greater possibilities for the provision of structures or toys within the pens. These can provide long-lasting interest for the dogs as well as allowing them to exercise some choice within the kennel environment. Some sites consider that toys are not worth the effort because of problems such as aggression or hygiene or lack of interest by the dogs. Appropriate presentation of the toys can overcome these objections, and dogs and puppies will make extensive use of toys or chews, particularly if they have an appetizing aroma (Hubrecht, 1993a, 1995a). In animal shelters, moreover, the presence of a toy within the pen can help to make a dog more attractive to prospective owners (Wells & Hepper, 1992). Groups of pens should be designed so that it is possible to move the animal to another pen temporarily during wet cleaning and so avoid exposing it to buckets of water, high-pressure hoses, and other aversive stimuli.

Visibility

Dogs have a natural interest in their surroundings, and kennels should not excessively restrict the dog's ability to obtain information about its surroundings. High walls or partitions between pens result in the inability of dogs to see the end of their rooms. This can lead to them spending a relatively high proportion of their time on hind legs or in apparently repetitive, possibly stereotypical, jumping behavior. Obvious ways around this problem include reducing solid partition height between pens or providing platforms within pens. Platforms are used extensively by dogs in laboratories to play and rest on (Hubrecht, 1993a). These structures increase the complexity of pens, thus allowing the dogs more choices within their environment, and provide a greater floor area within a given space. In effect, they make use of the otherwise neglected third dimension in the pen.

Dog housing should always be designed so that the dogs can retreat to an area that provides them with a sense of security. This need not cause a visibility problem for the caregiver. It can simply be an area with a few barriers shielding the animal from view on some sides. It is particularly important to provide such structures in large social groups to allow the dogs to control their social interactions.

Noise in Kennels

The noise in kennels resulting from barking can be a serious problem. Why dogs bark is not well understood, and dog vocalization behavior is different from that seen in wolves. Barking is not necessarily specific to particular contexts (Fox, 1971, 1978), although there is a strong territorial component. Barking in kennels often occurs when dogs bark at each other through adjacent pens or at people passing by the pens. Barking is also associated with the generally high levels of excitement at feeding times. Social facilitation often results in the barking spreading to other dogs (Fox, 1971). In some animals, the act of barking may act as a self-stimulus to further barking (Scott & Fuller, 1965).

Dogs can detect sounds ranging in frequency from 40 cycles per second (Hz) up to around 50 kHz, which is well beyond the upper frequency limit of human hearing. They are most sensitive to sounds at frequencies from 500 Hz to 16 kHz. In this range, their threshold of sensitivity can be 24 decibels (dB) lower than that of humans (Fay, 1988) so that they can hear sounds that are up to four times quieter than the human ear can detect. Noise levels in some kenneling are potentially damaging to human hearing and may constitute a nuisance to people living nearby (van der Heiden, 1992). Unfortunately, the possibility that the noise might have similar effects on dogs and their welfare has not been considered until recently. The noise problem for humans can be addressed by protective wear such as hearing defenders for the staff, but these are of no value to the dogs.

Sound levels within the human hearing range in dog kenneling can regularly reach values between 85 and 122 dB (Kay, 1972; Ottewill, 1968; Peterson, 1980), and similar levels have been reported for veterinary hospitals (Senn & Lewin, 1975). To assess the effects of their acoustic environment on the dogs, however, the total acoustic environment in which they live 24 hours a day must be known.

Summary: Dog Welfare

In most cases, the responsibilities and capabilities for ensuring that dog welfare is optimum are in human hands. Dogs do not have free will as to what use humans will make of them (i.e., companion animals, assistance dogs, service dogs, etc.) or of the conditions in which they are housed. Private and corporate owners, therefore, have a clear moral and, in some cases, legal responsibility for their dogs. Stray or feral dogs without an owner are the product of human actions; the responsibilities for these animals lie at a higher level with society.

Because of the wide variety of uses to which dogs are put, there are many potential situations in which their welfare may be compromised. Kenneling is an area with obvious gaps in knowledge of dogs' needs. Anyone designing a new kennel should take into account the considerations outlined above for appropriate kennel design, but it is also important to ensure that the kennel works as a whole and fulfills all the functions required of it. In most cases, sensible design and planning should allow the separate design requirements to be reconciled.

Good welfare means more than good physical health. The mental state of the animal must also be taken into account. An assessment of the dog with the five freedoms in mind will often suggest not only whether there is a problem but also the solution.

The Cat and Its Welfare

There are fewer studies of cat behavior welfare than those considering dogs. Only recently has the cat replaced the dog as the most popular companion animal in a number of countries, and interest in the domestic cat as a research subject has started to grow (Bradshaw, 1992; Turner, 1995a, 1995c; Turner & Bateson, 1988). The cat may also be more elusive, secretive, and less communicative than the dog (Bergler, 1986, 1989), adding to the difficulties of conducting research on this species.

Similarly to their application to dogs, the five freedoms (Farm Animal Welfare Council, 1993) can be used in any assessment of cat welfare under different housing situations. As for dogs, freedoms 1 (from thirst, hunger, and malnutrition) and 3 (from pain, injury, and disease) are relatively easy to control and provide for by proper husbandry and veterinary care of the cat. Most owners would agree on the status of animals observed. Obesity, however, can be an owner-caused problem in both species, the severity of which is judged differently among owners. Freedoms 2 (from discomfort) and 5 (from fear and distress) may be even more difficult for cat owners to assess because the cat appears to react differently from humans and human expectations based on other animals (McCune, 1992). For example, a stressed cat may simply move to the back of the cage and remain quiet, leading to the false interpretation of an adapted or relaxed cat. Freedom 4 (to express normal behavior) is perhaps less difficult to assess in cats than in dogs because of the relatively large number of feral and semiferal cat behavior studies that can be used as a reference system for behavior under other housing conditions (Turner, 1995b). Under the assumption that behavior regularly shown between cats and outside of the household is natural or normal, one can assess whether these patterns are shown (as frequently or without deviation) under various conditions of captivity. If not, or if they cannot be elicited by alternative stimuli or redirected to other objects, then those conditions might be detrimental to the animal. This approach to evaluating cat welfare will be taken below.

Cat Welfare in the Home

Having been domesticated for more than 3,500 years, cats are well adapted to living close to humans (Serpell, 1988). Their willingness to form close relationships with people and with other cats, however, depends on their socialization during the first weeks of life (Karsh & Turner, 1988; McCune, McPherson, & Bradshaw, 1995; Schär, 1989). Socialization to people and to conspecifics occurs independently and can take place simultaneously. If not properly socialized to the reference species with which they will later live, either the cats will not adapt and show signs of distress or the people will be disappointed, resulting in less harmonious relationships, possible broken bonds, and more stray animals (Kessler & Turner, 1995; Turner, 1995a, 1995c). In particular, social cats require contact with conspecifics (either indoors or outdoors), whereas solitary cats should not be forced to live indoors with other cats.

Cruelty and Neglect

Although every animal protection and welfare organization can provide a list of cases of deliberate cruelty to cats, unconscious cruelty is more frequent, while its consequences are less obvious. Cats have retained a high degree of independence despite domestication and are capable of hunting for their food, assuming prey animals are available in the area. Unfortunately, too many "problem" animals are permanently turned out onto the streets to fend for themselves, which often results in concentrations of free-ranging animals around food resources provided by humans (e.g., cat lovers and refuse dumps; Remfry, 1981). On the other hand, cats that are regularly allowed outdoor access can probably compensate for most mistakes people make in housing the animals (Turner, 1995a). Dogs are generally not allowed this freedom of movement but can at least compensate for any lack of exercise indoors during walks off the premises.

The question of maximum, let alone optimal, cat density in the private household is difficult to address. It is of utmost importance to animal welfare officers, however, who are regularly confronted with complaints about overpopulation (and possible mistreatment) in particular households. Unfortunately, there is only one study on the effects of cat density on animal stress, and that is in group housing in animal shelters (Kessler & Turner, 1996a). Experiences of pet behavior counselors and studies relating urine-marking behavior to group size in the private setting have led to a general rule of thumb: not more adult animals than the total number of rooms always available to the cats in that household (Turner, 1992). Of course, only cats socialized to conspecifics should be housed together.

Confinement

The issue of whether cats should be kept only indoors has become hotly contended in recent years. Two arguments are used by the proponents of banning cats from the outdoors: (a) to protect bird populations and (b) to protect cats from traffic dangers. There is no conclusive evidence of the endangerment of any endemic bird species principally by free-ranging cats on the continents, as opposed to the situation on small, offshore islands (Fitzgerald, 1988). The often cited Churcher and Lawton (1987) study in the United Kingdom is fraught with incorrect assumptions, and its conclusion is based on an incorrect extrapolation. This study did not juxtapose total predatory pressure against the total bird population, let alone consider the magnitude of normal yearly loss in any natural predator-prey system.

Although it is true that cats given access to the outdoors lead more dangerous lives and have a lower average life expectancy than do indoor cats, primarily because of traffic accidents, there is no evidence that their general welfare is lower than that of indoor cats. On the contrary, indoor cats are disproportionately more often represented among cats presented to pet behavior counselors with behavioral problems, most of which are related to improper housing conditions (Turner, 1995a). This is not to say that one cannot satisfy the welfare needs of cats indoors, but it does indicate that many owners of such cats do not. The biological and psychological needs of cats, as deduced from observations on (semi) free-ranging cats and from case studies in animal behavior clinics have been summarized (Turner, 1995a, 1995c). If these needs are not met, particularly when cats are kept exclusively indoors, detrimental effects can be expected on the animals' welfare. This can manifest itself in many ways, including reduced relationship quality, poor health, and behavioral disturbances (Turner, 1992, 1995a).

One aspect of confinement of cats indoors does require special mention, namely, the effects of confinement after a cat has gained experience outdoors. Again, on the basis of analysis of factors related to the appearance of behavioral problems in cats (Turner, 1995a), it behooves us to follow the general rule: Once an outdoor cat, always an outdoor cat! This should be taken into consideration when a move to a new abode is imminent and when shelters rehome animals.

Behavior Problems

Quite often, behavior problems are indicative of lower(ed) animal welfare. Domestic cats rarely show stereotypes but do react to improper housing conditions and changes in those conditions with "undesirable" behavior patterns (Turner, 1995a). The most frequent problems are urine marking (within the primary home), undesirable elimination, intraspecific aggression (within the group), claw sharpening away from the scratching post, pica (abnormal desire to eat unusual substances), and interspecific aggression toward the owner.

How seriously the welfare of the animal that shows one or more of these problems is jeopardized depends on the situation. Most problems can be successfully treated by properly trained advisers who investigate the proximate causes of the problem and propose either changes in the current housing conditions or behavior modification therapies (Turner, 1995a, 1997). Nevertheless, their importance to the animal's welfare should not be underestimated because many owners have reached the point of considering euthanasia if the problem cannot be solved.

Physical Problems

Artificial Selection

Fortunately, domestic cats have not been as intensively bred for as long as dogs, and until recently, most breeders have concentrated on appearance, especially coat color and hair characteristics, rather than on behavior, as has been the case with (working) dogs. Still, a number of problems have appeared (e.g., Persian cats with tear duct problems, lines that can bear young only with a cesarean section, and ear infections in breeds with folded pinea). Two recent "creations" are alarming (the hairless, or sphinx, cat and the Munchkin cat from the United States). The former is reportedly "ideal" for people allergic to cats, but the animal's welfare is compromised by thermoregulatory problems and the danger of direct sunlight. The Munchkin results in short, dachshund-like front legs and restrictions in the cat's ability to move about, particularly to jump. The mutation is dominant, and there is a danger that it might spread to other breeds, as well as to house cats. Anomalies and breed lines, which reduce the animals' welfare, making them incapable of survival without significant human intervention, should not be recognized by the breeder associations and should be prohibited by animal protection legislation in the future (Turner, 1996b).

Owner-Cat Matching

Although calls for optimal matching of people to cats have been made (Turner, 1984, 1991b, 1992; Turner & Stammbach-Geering, 1990), it is not possible to do so yet with any degree of reliability. The goals of such matching programs are to increase the probability of a harmonious relationship and lower the probability of later pet rejection. Hart and Hart (1985, 1995) have made a reasonable attempt to differentiate and classify the personality traits of dog breeds, and results have been reported of the first ethological study demonstrating differences in behavior and interactions with humans between three cat breeds (Siamese, Persian, and European shorthair cats; Turner, 1995a). These authors, however, were able to suggest only that future owners delve into their own personalities and consider their own desires and abilities to house specific breeds before selecting a particular animal (Turner, 1992, 1995c, 1996b). Some progress has been made in investigations of the relationship between owner personality and pet behavior and personality (Jagoe & Serpell, 1996; McBride & Cook, 1996; O'Farrell, 1997; Podberscek, 1996; Serpell, 1983, 1996; Turner, 1991b; Turner & Stammbach-Geering, 1990), but predictive results are not yet available. George and Kidd (1992) have at least been able to determine factors involved in explaining later pet rejection.

Ethical issues are involved in any attempt to "regulate," or even "steer," pet ownership on the basis of predictive tests of owner personality (Turner, 1996a) because a degree of uncertainty will always remain in factors explaining variance models. Nevertheless, such information could be used as a basis for discussion with potential owners and in designing educational programs to promote responsible pet ownership.

Cats in Institutions

Before addressing specifically the welfare of cats in shelters and asylums, in breeding catteries, and at cat exhibitions and in animal-assisted activity or therapy (AAA/AAT) programs, several general comments can be made about their housing and welfare in all institutions. The needs and requirements for proper housing of cats in institutions are the same as in private households (Turner, 1995c), but special attention must be paid to items of importance in institutional programs involving many animals and in which responsibility for care and welfare of the animals and people involved lies in the hands of the institution. First and foremost is proper veterinary examination and regular health controls, followed by registration (i.e., records) of the animals and attention to their social and spatial needs. In particular, stress to the animals is to be kept to a minimum (Kessler & Turner, 1996a, 1996b, in press; Smith, Durman, Roy, & Bradshaw, 1994).

Cats in Shelters and Asylums

Usually, the keeping of cats in shelters and asylums underlies animal protection/welfare laws, and it is important that those regulations be based on the most recent findings on the biological, psychological, and medicinal needs of cats. Private shelters and cat asylums (i.e., persons who take in a fairly large number of cats from the street and offer them shelter) are not always staffed by trained animal caretakers, and although their intentions are admirable, they deserve the same scrutiny as the shelters of acknowledged animal protection organizations. During peak holiday seasons, many shelters become filled, and it is important to see that (a) sufficient boarding places are available and (b) shelters do not become overfilled, lowering the individual animal's welfare during its stay (Kessler, in press; Kessler & Turner, 1995).

The social and spatial needs of cats admitted to and living in shelters and asylums should be met by the institution. Solitary cats should be kept alone in cages and pens, whereas social cats should be assigned to groups of other social cats, or at least kept together in pairs in sufficiently large enclosures. Tests have recently been refined to determine whether a homeless cat is solitary or social (Kessler & Turner, 1996b). Of course, facilities must be available to quarantine cats, although the procedure, especially when of a long duration, has significant short- and long-term effects on the behavior and temperament of cats and their behavior toward humans (Rochlitz, Podberscek, & Broom, 1996).

In shelters with group housing, attention must be paid to both the density of cats and the absolute number of cats in any one group to keep stress of the individuals to a minimum. With high use of the third dimension (cat shelves and climbing trees) and the possibility to build subgroups (e.g., the use of two connected rooms or enclosures), a maximum density of 1 cat per square meter and maximum total group size of 25 animals are recommended to inhibit the appearance of a despot in the group (Turner, 1992). A more recent recommendation is that cats in unstable groups (e.g., in shelters with changing group composition) have no less the 1.6 square meter of floor space, which results in only slight tension in the group (Kessler & Turner, 1996a).

Animal shelters usually attempt to rehome healthy animals, and some purport to see (and control) that the animals are placed in "good" homes. To date, only George and Kidd (1992) have presented results on factors affecting pet (not specifically cat) retention and rejection. Important adult predictors for retention were the adopter's age and expectations that the pet would be a playmate, companion, source of laughter, and provider of emotional support. Among the parents, the most important predictors for rejection were the expectations that the pets would keep the children busy and teach them love. As mentioned above, because of individual variation, it will always be impossible (and ethically questionable) to predict who will be a good or a bad adopter; it is probably safer and more correct to set (by law) or agree (by contract) to minimum standards for animal care and housing required to become an adopter.

Cats in Breeding Catteries and at Cat Exhibitions

The welfare of cats in breeding colonies is usually controlled by specifically designated persons in the cat breeders' associations. No published data are available on the results of such control visits, but it is probably safe to assume that the majority of cat breeders are indeed interested in the welfare of their animals, if only to protect their investment. Nevertheless, cases have appeared that are indicative of a lack (or disregard) of knowledge about the needs and welfare of the animals. It is important that breeders, especially those designated to control colonies, be well informed about those needs and cat welfare. Perhaps the best solution for the cats and breeders would be to set up, with the help of cat behavior experts and veterinarians, a list of minimum housing and care requirements and rules that must be met.

Cat exhibitions sometimes shock first-time visitors and must be designed in the future with more consideration of the cats' welfare (Turner, 1996b). Stress to the animals shown has never been measured, but it is conceivable that they adapt to the relatively small exhibition cages and handling by stewards and judges through time. Other potential problems at international cat shows include (a) the general noise level in the exhibition halls; (b) smoking, which is sometimes permitted; and (c) room temperature, which can become a problem to both the cats and the people present.

Cats in Animal-Assisted Activity or Therapy (AAA/AAT) Programs

These animals can generally be divided into two groups, residential and visitation animals. For cats, residential animals are more often involved. The ethical use of animals in such programs has recently been discussed (Turner, 1996a), with a conclusion that it is permissible under certain conditions. Those conditions include proper care and housing of the animals according to their needs, guarding against stress during transport and interactions (Iannuzzi & Rowan, 1991), and proper selection and training of both the animals and the people involved. The Delta Society (1992) of the United States has made an admirable first attempt to set guidelines for both AAA and AAT programs.

Summary: Cat Welfare

As in the case for dogs, the five freedoms may be applied to localize and solve the welfare problems of cats. Because cats are fairly adaptable to new situations and react differently from the expected (e.g., to stress), however, assessment of poor welfare in this species can be more elusive. Particular attention must be paid to housing the animals according to their degree of sociality, while still considering general recommendations on maximum density and absolute group size. Confinement indoors is discussed in connection with bird predation and traffic mortality, but it is argued that this may lead to behavioral disturbances if the cats cannot satisfy all their needs as determined from a reference system (i.e., the behavior of (semi-) free-ranging cats). Behavioral problems affect the quality of the owner's relationship with the cat, which in turn, affects the cat's welfare, especially when euthanasia is eminent. More research is required to predict optimal owner-cat matching.

Shelters and cat asylums must take into account the degree of sociality of their individual charges and of recent findings on maximum cat density and group size. Breeding associations and the organizers of cat shows must take on more responsibility in controlling for and promoting cat welfare. Programs involving cats in animal-assisted activities and therapy must safeguard the welfare of the animals and people involved.

Conclusion

Interactions and relationships with both cats and dogs must, in the end, be guided by two principles: responsible ownership and responsible trusteeship. Once people realize that these animals have their own needs and requirements and respect those in dealing with them, the welfare of all parties involved will be maintained, and in many cases improved, and both humans and animals will benefit from these social partnerships.

References

Anderson, R. K., Hart, B. & Hart, L. (Eds.). (1984). *The pet connection*. Minneapolis: University of Minnesota, CENSHARE.

Bergler, R. (1986). *Man and dog: Psychology of a relationship*. Oxford, UK: Blackwell Scientific.

Bergler, R. (1989). *Man and cat: The benefits of cat ownership*. Oxford, UK: Blackwell Scientific.

Blythe, L. L., Gannon, J. R., & Craig, A. M. (1994). *Care of the racing greyhound: A guide for trainers, breeders and veterinarians*. Portland, OR: Graphic Arts Center.

Bonner, J. (1995, September 30). Off with their tails. *New Scientist, 16-17.*

Bradshaw, J. W. S. (1992). *The behavior of the domestic cat.* Wallingford, UK: CAB International.

Bradshaw, J. W. S., & Brown, S. (1990). Behavioral adaptations of dogs to domestication. *Waltham Symposium, 20,* 18-24.

Bradshaw, J. W. S., Goodwin, D., Lea, A. M., & Whitehead, S. L. (1996). A survey of behavioral characteristics of pure-bred dogs in the United Kingdom. *Veterinary Record, 138,* 465-468.

Churcher, P. B., & Lawton, J. H. (1987). Predation by domestic cats in an English village. *Journal of Zoology, London, 212,* 439-455.

Clark, J. D., Calpin, J. P., & Armstrong, R. B. (1991). Influence of type of enclosure on exercise fitness of dogs. *American Journal of Veterinary Research, 52,* 1024-1028.

Clutton-Brock, J. (1995). Origins of the dog: Domestication and early history. In J. Serpell (Ed.), *The domestic dog: Its evolution, behavior and interactions with people* (pp. 7-20). Cambridge, UK: Cambridge University Press.

Coppinger, R. (1995). *Wheelchair assistance dogs.* Amherst MA: Hampshire College, Dog Studies Program and Lemelson Center for Assistive Technology Development.

Coppinger, R., & Schneider, R. (1995). Evolution of working dogs. In J. Serpell (Ed.), *The domestic dog: Its evolution, behavior and interactions with people* (pp. 21-47). Cambridge, UK: Cambridge University Press.

Delta Society. (1992). *Handbook for animal-assisted activities and animal-assisted therapy.* Renton, WA: Author.

Farm Animal Welfare Council. (1993). *Second report on priorities for animal welfare research and development in farm animal welfare.* Tolworth, UK: MAFF.

Fay, R. (1988). *Hearing in vertebrates: A psychophysics data book.* Winnetka, IL: Hill-Fay.

Fitzgerald, B. M. (1988). Diet of domestic cats and their impact on prey populations. In D. C. Turner & P. Bateson (Eds.), *The domestic cat: The biology of its behavior* (pp. 159-178). Cambridge, UK: Cambridge University Press.

Fogle, B. (Ed.). (1981). *Interrelations between people and pets.* Springfield, IL: Charles C Thomas.

Fox, M. W. (1971). *Behavior of wolves, dogs and related canids.* London: Jonathan Cape.

Fox, M. W. (1978). *The dog: Its domestication and behavior.* New York: Garland STPM.

George, C. C., & Kidd, A. H. (1992, July). *Using the pet expectations inventory to predict pet rejection.* Paper presented at the International Society of Anthrozoology Symposium, Montreal, Quebec, Canada.

Hart, B. L., & Hart, L. A. (1985). *Canine and feline behavioral therapy.* Philadelphia: Lea & Febiger.

Hart, B. L., & Hart, L. A. (1995). *The perfect puppy.* New York: Freeman.

Hetts, S. (1991): Psychologic well-being: Conceptual issues, behavioral measures and implications for dogs. *Advances in Companion Animal Behavior, 21,* 369-387.

Hubrecht, R. C. (1993a) A comparison of social and environmental enrichment methods for laboratory housed dogs. *Applied Animal Behavior Science, 37,* 345-361.

Hubrecht, R. C. (1993b). *Dog housing and welfare* (UFAW Animal Research Report No. 6). Potters Bar, UK: Universities Federation for Animal Welfare.

Hubrecht, R. C. (1995a). Enrichment in puppyhood and its effect on later behavior of dogs. *Laboratory Animal Science, 45,* 70-75.

Hubrecht, R. C. (1995b). The welfare of dogs in human care. In J. Serpell (Ed.), *The domestic dog: Evolution, behaviour, and interactions with people* (pp. 179-198). Cambridge, UK: Cambridge University Press.

Hubrecht, R. C., Serpell, J. A., & Poole T. B. (1992). Correlates of pen size and housing conditions on the behavior of kennelled dogs. *Applied Animal Behavior Science, 34,* 365-383.

Iannuzzi, D., & Rowan, A. N. (1991). Ethical issues in animal-assisted therapy programs. *Anthrozoös, 4,* 154-163.

IEMT. (Ed.). (1985). *The human pet relationship: Essays on the occasion of the 80th birthday of Nobel prize laureate professor Dr. Konrad Lorenz.* Vienna: Austrian Academy of Science.

Jagoe, A., & Serpell, J. A. (1996). Owner characteristics and interactions and the prevalence of canine behavior problems. *Applied Animal Behavior Science, 47,* 31-42.

Karsh, E. B., & Turner, D. C. (1988). The human-cat relationship. In D. C. Turner & P. Bateson (Eds.), *The domestic cat: The biology of its behavior* (pp. 159-178). Cambridge, UK: Cambridge University Press.

Katcher, A. H., & Beck, A. M. (Eds.). (1983). *New perspectives on our lives with companion animals.* Philadelphia: University of Pennsylvania Press.

Kay, R. S. (1972). *The construction of a small-animal hospital: An investigation into problems involved with special reference to noise.* Unpublished thesis, Royal College of Veterinary Surgeons, Cambridge, UK.

Kessler, M. (in press). *Erhebung zur bestehenden Haltungssituation für Katzen (Felis catus) in deutschschweizer Tierheimen* [Analysis of the current housing situation for cats in animal shelters of German-speaking Switzerland]. *Swiss Archive for Veterinary Medicine (SAT).*

Kessler, M., & Turner, D. C. (1995). *Katzenhaltung im Tierheim: Analyse der bestehenden Haltungssituation für Katzen in deutschschweizer Tierheimen* [Cats in animal shelters: An analysis of the current situation in shelters of German-speaking Switzerland]. Zurich, Switzerland: Zürcher Tierschutz.

Kessler, M., & Turner, D. C. (1996a). *Effects of density and cage size on stress in domestic cats housed in animal shelters and boarding catteries.* Manuscript submitted for publication.

Kessler, M., & Turner, D. C. (1996b). *Socialization and stress in domestic cats housed singly and in groups in animal shelters.* Manuscript submitted for publication.

Kessler, M., & Turner, D. C. (in press). Stress and adaptation of cats (Felis silvestris catus) housed singly, in pairs and in groups in boarding catteries. *Animal Welfare.*

Ledger, R., Baxter, M., & McNicholas, J. (1995). Temperament testing dogs in a rescue shelter: Improving dog-owner compatibility. In S. M. Rutter, J. Rushen, H. D. Randle, & J. C. Eddison (Eds.), *Proceedings of the 29th International Congress of the ISAE* (pp. 101-102). Potters Bar, UK: Universities Federation for Animal Welfare.

MacArthur, J. A. (1987). The dog. In T. Poole (Ed.), *The UFAW handbook on the care and management of laboratory animals* (6th ed., pp. 456-475). Harlow, UK: Longman.

McBride, E. A., & Cook, S. E. (1996). Relationship between personality traits and attitudes to cats in members of cat-owning households [Abstract]. In A. Podberscek (Ed.), *International Society of Anthrozoology abstracts: The animal contract.* Cambridge, UK: Downing College.

McCune, S. (1992). *Temperament and welfare of caged cats.* Unpublished doctoral dissertation, University of Cambridge, Cambridge, UK.

McCune, S., McPherson, J. A., & Bradshaw, J. W. S. (1995). Avoiding problems: The importance of socialisation. In I. Robinson (Ed.), *The Waltham book of human-animal interaction: Benefits and responsibilities of pet ownership* (pp. 71-86). Oxford, UK: Pergamon.

O'Farrell, V. (1997). Owner attitudes and dog behavior problems. In D. C. Turner (Ed.), Behavioral problems of small animals [Special issue]. *Applied Animal Behavior Science.*

Ottewill, D. (1968). Planning and design of accommodation for experimental dogs and cats. *Laboratory Animal Symposium, 1,* 97-112.

Peterson, E. A. (1980). Noise and laboratory animals. *Laboratory Animal Science, 30,* 422-439.

Podberscek, A. (1996). Yikes! Owner personality and aggressive behavior in English cocker spaniels [Abstract]. In A. Podberscek (Ed.), *International Society of Anthrozoology abstracts: The animal contract.* Cambridge, UK: Downing College.

Remfry, J. (1981). Strategies for control. In Universities Federation for Animal Welfare (Ed.), *The ecology and control of feral cats.* Potters Bar, UK: Universities Federation for Animal Welfare.

Rochlitz, I., Podberscek, A. & Broom, D. M. (1996). The effects of quarantine on cats: Owners' reports. [Abstract]. In A. Podberscek (Ed.), *International Society of Anthrozoology abstracts: The animal contract.* Cambridge, UK: Downing College.

Rowan, A. N. (Ed.). (1988). *Animals and people sharing the world.* Hanover, NH: Universities Press of New England.

Sargan, D. R. (1995). Research in canine and human genetic disease [Conference report]. *Journal of Medical Genetics, 32,* 751-754.

Schär, R. (1989). *Die Hauskatze: Lebensweise und Ansprüche* [The house cat: Its lifestyle and requirements]. Stuttgart, Germany: Verlag Eugen Ulmer.

Scott, J. P., & Fuller, J. L. (1965). *Genetics and social behavior of the dog.* Chicago: University of Chicago Press.

Senn, C. L., & Lewin, J. D. (1975). Barking dogs as an environmental problem. *Journal of the American Veterinary Medical Association, 166,* 1065-1068.

Serpell, J. A. (1983). The personality of the dog and its influence on the pet-owner bond. In A. H. Katcher & A. M. Beck (Eds.), *New perspectives on our lives with companion animals* (pp. 57-65). Philadelphia: University of Pennsylvania Press.

Serpell, J. A. (1988). The domestication of the cat. In D. C. Turner & P. Bateson (Eds.), *The domestic cat: The biology of its behavior* (pp. 151-158). Cambridge, UK: Cambridge University Press.

Serpell, J. A. (1996). Evidence for an association between pet behavior and owner attachment levels. *Applied Animal Behavior Science, 47,* 49-60.

Serpell, J. A., & Jagoe, J. A. (1995). Early experience and the development of behavior. In J. Serpell (Ed.), *The domestic dog: Its evolution, behavior and interactions with people* (pp. 79-102). Cambridge, UK: Cambridge University Press.

Smith, D. F. E., Durman, K. J., Roy, D. B., & Bradshaw, J. W. S. (1994). Behavioral aspects of the welfare of rescued cats. *Journal of the Feline Advisory Bureau, 31,* 25-28.

Turner, D. C. (1984). Overview of research on human-animal interaction in Switzerland. *Journal of the Delta Society, 1,* 44-45.

Turner, D. C. (1991a). Ethologie und die Mensch-Tier Beziehung [The ethology of the human-animal relationship]. In H. Holzhey & A. Rust (Eds.), *Ethische Konflikte in der Tiernutzung* [Ethical conflicts in the use of animals] (pp. 32-40). Zurich, Switzerland: Philosophisches Seminar der Universität Zürich.

Turner, D. C. (1991b). The ethology of the human-cat relationship. *Schweizer Archiv für Tierheilkunde, 133,* 63-70.

Turner, D. C. (1992). *Von Katzen und Menschen* [On cats and people]. Zurich, Switzerland: Zürcher Tierschutz.

Turner, D. C. (1995a). *Die Mensch-Katze Beziehung: Ethologische und psychologische Aspekte* [The human-cat relationship: Ethological and psychological aspects]. Jena, Germany: Gustav Fischer Verlag.

Turner, D. C. (1995b). Ethologie und Wohlbefinden der Heimtiere [Ethology and companion animal welfare]. *Schweizer Archiv für Tierheilkunde, 137,* 45-49

Turner, D. C. (1995c). The human-cat relationship. In I. Robinson (Ed.), *The Waltham book of human-animal interaction: Benefits and responsibilities of pet ownership* (pp. 87-97). Oxford, UK: Pergamon.

Turner, D. C. (1996a). Ethical issues in companion animal ownership, use and research. In J. Nicholson & A. Podberscek (Eds.), *Further issues in research in companion animal studies* (Vol. 3). Callander, Scotland: Society for Companion Animal Studies.

Turner, D. C. (1996b). *Katzen lieben und verstehen* [Loving and understanding cats]. Stuttgart, Germany: Franckh-Kosmos Verlag and Tokyo: Pet Life Sha.

Turner, D. C. (1997). Treating canine and feline behavior problems and advising clients. In D. C. Turner (Ed.), Behavioral problems of small animals [Special issue]. *Applied Animal Behavior Science.*

Turner, D. C. & Bateson, P. (Eds.). (1988). *The domestic cat: The biology of its behavior.* Cambridge, UK: Cambridge University Press.

Turner, D. C., & Stammbach-Geering, K. B. (1990). Owner assessment and the ethology of human-cat relationships. In I. Burger (Ed.), *Pets, benefits and practice* (pp. 25-30). London: British Veterinary Association.

van der Heiden, C. V. (1992): The problem of noise within kennels: What are its implications and how can it be reduced? *Veterinary Nursing Journal, 7,* 13-16.

Vincent, I. C. (1993): Is there a link between behavior and blood pressure in dogs? *Veterinary Nursing Journal, 8,* 43-45.

Webster, J. (1994). *Eden animal welfare: A cool eye towards Eden.* Oxford, UK: Blackwell Science.

Wells, D., & Hepper, P. G. (1992): The behavior of dogs in a rescue shelter. *Animal Welfare, 1,* 171-186.

Wickens, S. M., Astell-Billings, I., McPherson, J. A., Gibb, R., Bradshaw, J. W. S., & McBride, E. A. (1995). The behavioral assessment of dogs in animal shelters: Interobserver reliability and data redundancy. In S. M. Rutter, J. Rushen, H. D. Randle, & J. C. Eddison (Eds.), *Proceedings of the 29th International Congress of the ISAE* (pp. 101-102). Potters Bar, UK: Universities Federation for Animal Welfare.

Willis, M. B. (1995): Genetic aspects of dog behavior with particular reference to working ability. In J. Serpell (Ed.), *The domestic dog: Its evolution, behavior and interactions with people* (pp. 51-64). Cambridge, UK: Cambridge University Press.

Index

About the Editors

Cindy C. Wilson, Ph.D., C.H.E.S., received her B.S. in microbiology, her M.S. in animal science and statistics, and her Ph.D. in public health from the University of Tennessee. She is currently Professor and Faculty Development Director for Family Medicine programs through the Uniformed Services University of the Health Sciences in Bethesda, Maryland. She has research and practice experience in gerontological programs as well as in pet placement and visitation programs. She presented her research in the area of physiological and psychologic responses of college students to a pet at the National Institutes of Health Technology Assessment Conference in 1987 and continues to publish data-based as well as conceptual projects on therapeutic uses of human-animal interventions. In addition to her work on quality of life and clinical trials, she has served on the editorial board of *Anthrozoös* for many years and serves as a reviewer for four other major health journals. She continues to conduct her own research in a wide range of topic areas and to support the work of faculty colleagues at the military Family Medicine sites worldwide. She serves as a consultant to a number of businesses and university programs in the area of research design and methodology.

Dennis C. Turner, B.S., Sc.D., received his B.S. in biology from San Diego State University and his doctorate in animal behavior and ecology from Johns Hopkins University School of Hygiene and Public Health in Baltimore. He is currently a tenured lecturer at the University of Zurich, Director of the private scientific Institute for Applied Ethology and Animal Psychology, President of the Konrad Lorenz Trust-IEMT in Switzerland, and President of the International Association of Human-Animal Interaction Organizations, I.A.H.A.I.O. His research concerns cat and dog behavior and the ethology and psychology of human-cat relations. He is European editor of the journal *Anthrozoös* and companion animal section editor of the journal *Animal Welfare*. He has authored several books and is coeditor (with Patrick Bateson) of *The Domestic Cat: The Biology of Its Behaviour.*

About the Contributors

Warwick P. Anderson is with the Alfred and Baker Medical Unit, Baker Medical Research Institute, WHO Collaborating Center for Research and Training in Cardiovascular Disease, Prahran, Victoria, Australia.

Ivan Barofsky, Ph.D., is Associate Professor of Medical Psychology with the Pain and Work Rehabilitation Clinic at Johns Hopkins Bayview Medical Center in Baltimore, Maryland.

Kathryn Batson, M.S.N., is a former graduate student from the University of Nebraska Medical Center, College of Nursing, Omaha.

Mara M. Baun, D.N.Sc., F.A.A.N., is a professor at the University of Nebraska Medical Center, College of Nursing, Omaha.

Reinhold Bergler, Ph.D., is with the Institute der Stiftung für empirische Sozialforschung in Nuremberg, Germany.

Nancy M. Bodmer, M.Sc., specialized in developmental psychology at the Institute of Psychology, University of Berne, Switzerland.

Leo K. Bustad, Ph.D., DVM, is Dean Emeritus at the College of Veterinary Medicine, Washington State University, Pullman.

Glyn M. Collis, B.Sc., Ph.D., is Director of Postgraduate Studies in Psychology in the Department of Psychology of the University of Warwick, Coventry, England.

Jane Copeland Fitzpatrick, B.Sc., M.A., is Executive Director of Pegasus Therapeutic Riding and Physical Therapist in Darien, Connecticut.

Irene Christy is with the Alfred and Baker Medical Unit, Baker Medical Research Institute, WHO Collaborating Center for Research and Training in Cardiovascular Disease, Prahran, Victoria, Australia.

Anthony Dart is with the Alfred and Baker Medical Unit, Baker Medical Research Institute, WHO Collaborating Center for Research and Training in Cardiovascular Disease, Prahran, Victoria, Australia.

Susan L. Duncan, R.N., is Health Care Education Specialist and Coordinator for the Delta Society National Service Dog Center in Renton, Washington.

Maureen Fredrickson, MSW, is Program Director of the Delta Society in Renton, Washington.

Erika Friedmann, Ph.D., is Professor and Chairperson, Department of Health and Nutrition Sciences, Brooklyn College of CUNY, New York.

Thomas F. Garrity, Ph.D., is Chairman and Professor of the Department of Behavioral Science, College of Medicine, at the University of Kentucky in Lexington.

Linda Hines is President/CEO of the Delta Society in Renton, Washington.

Robert Hubrecht, Ph.D., is with the Universities Federation for Animal Welfare, Potters Bar, Herts, England.

Garry L. R. Jennings, Ph.D. or M.D., is Professor at the Heart Centre at Alfred Hospital and Director of the Alfred and Baker Medical Unit, Baker Medical Research Institute, WHO Collaborating Center for Research and Training in Cardiovascular Disease, Prahran, Victoria, Australia.

Janis Jennings is with the Alfred and Baker Medical Unit, Baker Medical Research Institute, WHO Collaborating Center for Research and Training in Cardiovascular Disease, Prahran, Victoria, Australia.

Carolyn P. Keil, R.N., Ph.D., is on the faculty of the School of Nursing at the University of Alaska in Anchorage.

Barbara McCabe, Ph.D., R.N., is an associate professor at the University of Nebraska Medical Center, College of Nursing, Omaha.

June McNicholas, B.Sc., is with the Department of Psychology of the University of Warwick, Coventry, England.

Gail F. Melson, Ph.D., is Professor of Child Development and Family Studies at Purdue Univrsity, West Lafayette, Indiana.

Christopher M. Reid is with the Alfred and Baker Medical Unit, Baker Medical Research Institute, WHO Collaborating Center for Research and Training in Cardiovascular Disease, Prahran, Victoria, Australia.

Andrew Rowan, Ph.D., was Editor-in-Chief of the journal *Anthrozoös* and is on the faculty of the School of Veterinary Medicine at Tufts University, North Grafton, Massachusetts, and Assistant Dean for new programs. He is now Vice President for the Humane Society of the U.S.

Lorann Stallones, Ph.D., is Professor in the Department of Environmental Health, College of Veterinary Medicine and Biomedical Sciences, Colorado State University, Fort Collins.

Melanie C. Steffens is with the Institute of Psychology at the University Trier in Trier, Germany.

Jean M. Tebay, B.A., M.S., is Director of Therapeutic Riding Services in Lutherville, Maryland.

310 COMPANION ANIMALS IN HUMAN HEALTH

Sue A. Thomas, R.N., Ph.D., is Executive Director of New Life Directions in Ellicott City, Maryland.

Sandra Lookabaugh Triebenbacher, Ph.D., is Assistant Professor in the Department of Child Development and Family Relations of East Carolina University, Greenville, North Carolina.

Carol Wilson, R.N., M.S.N., is the retired Director of Nursing of the University Hospital and a clinical associate of the University of Nebraska Medical Center, College of Nursing, Omaha.